THE
FastDiet

THE
FastDiet

Lose Weight, Stay Healthy, and
Live Longer with the Simple Secret
of Intermittent Fasting

Dr. Michael Mosley
Mimi Spencer

ATRIA BOOKS

New York   London   Toronto   Sydney   New Delhi

This publication contains the opinions and ideas of its author. It is intended to provide helpful and informative material on the subjects addressed in the publication. It is sold with the understanding that the author and publisher are not engaged in rendering medical, health, or any other kind of personal or professional services in the book. The reader should consult his or her medical, health, or other competent professional before adopting any of the suggestions in this book or drawing inferences from it.

The author and publisher specifically disclaim all responsibility for any liability, loss, or risk, personal or otherwise, which is incurred as a consequence, directly or indirectly, of the use and applications of any of the contents of this book.

ATRIA BOOKS
A Division of Simon & Schuster, Inc.
1230 Avenue of the Americas
New York, NY 10020

Copyright © 2013 by Dr. Michael Mosley and Mimi Spencer

All rights reserved, including the right to reproduce this book or portions thereof in any form whatsoever. For information, address Atria Books Subsidiary Rights Department, 1230 Avenue of the Americas, New York, NY 10020.

First Atria Books hardcover edition February 2013

ATRIA BOOKS and colophon are trademarks of Simon & Schuster, Inc.

For information about special discounts for bulk purchases, please contact Simon & Schuster Special Sales at 1-866-506-1949 or business@simonandschuster.com.

The Simon & Schuster Speakers Bureau can bring authors to your live event. For more information or to book an event, contact the Simon & Schuster Speakers Bureau at 1-866-248-3049 or visit our website at www.simonspeakers.com.

Designed by Kyoko Watanabe

Food photography by Romas Foord

Manufactured in the United States of America

10 9 8

Library of Congress Cataloging-in-Publication Data
Mosley, Michael.
  The fastdiet : lose weight, stay healthy, and live longer with the simple secret of intermittent fasting / Dr. Michael Mosley and Mimi Spencer.
    pages   cm
    Includes bibliographical references and index.
  1. Reducing diets—Recipes. 2. Diet. I. Spencer, Mimi. II. Title.
  RM222.2.M652   2013
  613.2'5—dc23   2012049657

ISBN 978-1-4767-3494-1
ISBN 978-1-4767-3496-5 (ebook)

*For my wife, Clare, and children, Alex, Jack, Daniel,
and Kate, who make living longer worthwhile.*

—M.M.

*For Ned, Lily May, and Paul—my Brighton rock. And for
my parents, who have always known that food is love.*

—M.S.

Contents

THE
FastDiet

Introduction

OVER THE LAST FEW DECADES, FOOD FADS HAVE come and gone, but the standard medical advice on what constitutes a healthy lifestyle has stayed much the same: eat low-fat foods, exercise more . . . and never, ever skip meals. Over that same period, levels of obesity worldwide have soared.

So is there a different evidence-based approach? One that relies on science, not opinion? Well, we think there is: intermittent fasting.

When we first read about the alleged benefits of intermittent fasting, we, like many, were skeptical. Fasting seemed drastic, difficult—and we both knew that dieting of any description is generally doomed to fail. But now that we've looked at it in depth and tried it ourselves, we are convinced of its remarkable potential. As one of the medical experts

> There is nothing else you can do to your body that is as powerful as fasting.

interviewed for this book puts it: "There is nothing else you can do to your body that is as powerful as fasting."

Fasting: An Ancient Idea, a Modern Method

Fasting is nothing new. As we'll discover in the next chapter, your body is designed to fast. We evolved at a time when food was scarce; we are the product of millennia of feast or famine. The reason we respond so well to intermittent fasting may be because it mimics, far more accurately than three meals a day, the environment in which modern humans were shaped.

Fasting, of course, remains an article of faith for many. The fasts of Lent, Yom Kippur, and Ramadan are just some of the better-known examples. Greek Orthodox Christians are encouraged to fast for 180 days of the year (according to Saint Nikolai of Zicha, "Gluttony makes a man gloomy and fearful, but fasting makes him joyful and courageous"), while Buddhist monks fast on the new moon and full moon of each lunar month.

Many more of us, however, seem to be eating most of the time. We're rarely ever hungry. But we *are* dissatisfied. With our weight, our bodies, our health.

Intermittent fasting can put us back in touch with our human selves. It is a route not only to weight loss, but also to long-term health and well-being. Scientists are only just beginning to discover and prove how powerful a tool it can be.

This book is a product of those scientists' cutting-edge investigations and their impact on our current thinking about weight loss, disease resistance, and longevity. But it is also the result of our personal experiences.

Both are relevant here—the lab and the lifestyle—so we investigate intermittent fasting from two complementary perspectives. First, Michael, who used his body and medical training to test its potential, explains the scientific foundations of intermittent fasting (IF) and the 5:2 diet—something he brought to the world's attention during the summer of 2012.

Then Mimi offers a practical guide on how to do it safely, effectively, and in a sustainable way, a way that will fit easily into your normal everyday life. She looks in detail at how fasting feels, what you can expect from day to day, what to eat, and when to eat, and provides a host of tips and strategies to help you gain the greatest benefit from the diet's simple precepts.

As you'll see below, the FastDiet has changed both of our lives. We hope it will do the same for you.

Michael's Motivation: A Male Perspective

I am a 55-year-old male, and before I embarked on my exploration of intermittent fasting, I was mildly overweight: at five feet, eleven inches, I weighed around 187 pounds and had a body mass index of 26, which put me into the overweight category. Until my midthirties, I had been slim, but

3

like many people I then gradually put on weight, around one pound a year. This doesn't sound like much, but over a couple of decades it pushed me up and up. Slowly I realized that I was starting to resemble my father, a man who struggled with weight all his life and died in his early seventies of complications associated with diabetes. At his funeral many of his friends commented on how like him I had become.

While making a documentary for the BBC, I was fortunate enough to have an MRI (magnetic resonance imaging) scan done. This revealed that I am a TOFI—thin on the outside, fat inside. This visceral fat is the most dangerous sort of fat, because it wraps itself around your internal organs and puts you at risk for heart disease and diabetes. I later had blood tests that showed I was heading toward diabetes, and had a cholesterol score that was also way too high. Obviously, I was going to have to do something about this. I tried following standard advice, except it made little difference. My weight and blood profile remained stuck in the "danger ahead" zone.

I had never tried dieting before because I'd never found a diet that I thought would work. I'd watched my father try every form of diet, from Scarsdale through Atkins, from the Cambridge Diet to the Drinking Man's Diet. He'd lost weight on each one of them, and then within a few months put it all back on, and more.

Then, at the beginning of 2012, I was approached by Aidan Laverty, editor of the BBC science series *Horizon*, who asked if I would like to put myself forward as a guinea pig to explore the science behind life extension. I wasn't sure what we would find, but along with producer Kate Dart and researcher Roshan Samarasinghe, we quickly focused on calorie restriction and fasting as a fruitful area to explore.

Calorie restriction (CR) is pretty brutal; it involves eating an awful lot less than a normal person would expect to eat, and doing so every day of your (hopefully) long life. The reason people put themselves through this is because it is the only intervention that has been shown to extend lifespan, at least in animals. There are at least 10,000 CRONies (Calorie Restriction with Optimum Nutrition) worldwide, and I have met quite a number of them. Despite their generally fabulous biochemical profile, I have never been seriously tempted to join their skinny ranks. I simply don't have the willpower or desire to live permanently on an extreme low-calorie diet.

So I was delighted to discover intermittent fasting (IF), which involves eating fewer calories, but *only some of the time*. If the science was right, it offered the benefits of CR but without the pain.

I set off around the United States, meeting leading scientists who generously shared their research and ideas with me. It became clear that IF was no fad. But it wouldn't be as easy as I'd originally hoped. As you'll see later in the book, there are many different forms of intermittent fasting. Some involve eating nothing for twenty-four hours or longer. Others involve eating a single, low-calorie meal once a day, every other day. I tried both but couldn't imagine doing either on a regular basis. I found it was simply too hard.

Instead I decided to create and test my own modified version. Five days a week, I would eat normally; on the remaining two I would eat a quarter of my usual calorie intake (that is, 600 calories).

I split the 600 calories in two—around 250 calories for breakfast and 350 calories for supper—effectively fasting for around twelve hours at a stretch. I also decided to split my fasting days: I would fast on Mondays and Thursdays. I became my own experiment.

The program, *Eat, Fast, Live Longer*, which detailed my adventures with what we were now calling the 5:2 diet, appeared on the BBC during the London Olympics in August 2012. I expected it to be lost in the media frenzy that surrounded the Games, but instead it generated a frenzy of its own. The program was watched by more than 2.5 million people—a huge audience for *Horizon*—and hundreds of thousands more on YouTube. My Twitter account went into overdrive, my followers tripled; everyone wanted to try my version of intermittent fasting, and they were all asking me what they should do.

The newspapers took up the story. Articles appeared in *The Times* (London), the *Daily Telegraph*, the *Daily Mail*, and the *Mail on Sunday*. Before long, it was picked up by newspapers all over the world—in New York, Los Angeles, Paris, Madrid, Montreal, Islamabad, and New Delhi. Online groups were created, menus and experiences swapped, chat rooms started buzzing about fasting. People began to stop me on the street and tell me how well they were doing on the 5:2 diet. They also e-mailed details of their experiences. Among those e-mails, a surprisingly large number were from doctors. Like me, they had initially been skeptical, but they had tried it for themselves, found that it worked, and had begun suggesting it to their patients. They wanted information, menus, details of the scientific research to scrutinize. They wanted me to write a book. I hedged, procrastinated, then finally found a collaborator, Mimi Spencer, whom I liked and trusted and who has an in-depth knowledge of food. Which is how what you are reading came about.

Michael's Background

I trained as a doctor at the Royal Free Hospital in London, and after passing my medical exams, I joined the BBC as a trainee assistant producer. Over the last twenty-five years, I have made numerous science and history documentaries for the BBC, first behind the camera, more recently in front. I was executive producer of *QED*; *Trust Me, I'm a Doctor*; and *Superhuman*. I worked with John Cleese, Jeremy Clarkson, Professor Robert Winston, Sir David Attenborough, and Professor Alice Roberts. I devised and executive-produced many programs for the BBC and the Discovery Channel, including: *Pompeii: The Last Day, Supervolcano*, and *Krakatoa: Volcano of Destruction*.

As a presenter I have made a dozen series for the BBC, including *Medical Mavericks, Blood and Guts, Inside Michael Mosley, Science Story, The Young Ones, Inside the Human Body*, and *The Truth About Exercise*. I am currently making three new series, as well as being a regular science presenter for the BBC's *The One Show*.

I have won numerous awards, including being named Medical Journalist of the Year by the British Medical Association.

Mimi's Motivation: A Female Perspective

I started intermittent fasting on the day I was commissioned to write a feature for *The Times* about Michael's *Horizon* program. It was the first I'd heard of intermittent fasting, and the idea appealed immediately, even to a cynical soul who has spent two decades examining the curious acrobatics of the fashion industry, the beauty business, and the diet trade.

I'd dabbled in diets before—show me a fortysomething woman who hasn't—losing weight, then losing faith within weeks and piling it all back on. Though never overweight, I'd long been interested in dropping that reluctant seven to ten pounds—the pounds I picked up in pregnancy and somehow never lost. The diets I tried were always too hard to follow, too complicated to implement, too boring, too tough, too single-strand, too invasive, sucking the juice out of life and leaving you with the scraps. There was nothing I found that I could adopt and thread into the context of my life—as a mother, a working woman, a wife.

I've argued for years that dieting is a fool's game, doomed to fail because of the restrictions and deprivations imposed on an otherwise happy life, but this felt immediately differ-ent. The scientific evidence was extensive and compelling, and (crucially for me) the medical community was positive. The effects, for Michael and others, were impressive, star-tling even. In his *Horizon* documentary, Michael called it the "beginning of something huge . . . which could radically transform the nation's health." I couldn't resist. Nor could I conceive of a reason to wait.

> The scientific evidence was extensive and compelling, and (crucially for me) the medical community was positive.

In the months since I wrote the *Times* feature, I have re-mained a convert. An evangelist, actually. I'm still "on" the FastDiet now, but I barely notice it. At the outset, I weighed 132 pounds. At five feet, seven inches, my BMI was an okay 21.4. Today, as I write, I weigh 119 pounds, with a BMI of 19.4. That's a weight off. I feel light, lean, and alive. Fasting has become part of my weekly life, something I do auto-matically without stressing about it.

Six months in, I have more en-ergy, more bounce, clearer skin, a greater zest for life. And—it has to be said—new jeans (27-inch waist) and none of my annual bikini dread as summer ap-proaches. But perhaps more important, I know that there's

> I feel light, lean, and alive.

a long-term gain. I'm doing the best for my body and my brain. It's an intimate revelation, but one worth sharing.

Mimi's Background

I have written about fashion, food, and body shape in British national newspapers and magazines for twenty years, starting out at *Vogue*, followed by *The Guardian*, *The Observer*, and the *London Evening Standard*, where I was named British Fashion Journalist of the Year in 2000. I am currently a columnist for the *Mail on Sunday*'s *You* magazine and a regular features writer for *The Saturday Times*. In 2009 I wrote a book, *101 Things to Do Before You Diet*, cataloguing my dismay with fad diets, which seem forever doomed to fail. Intermittent fasting is the only plan I have discovered in two decades that gets the weight off and keeps it off. And the antiaging health benefits? Gravy.

The FastDiet: The Potential, the Promise

We know that for many people, the standard diet advice simply does not work. The FastDiet is a radical alternative. It has the potential to change the way we think about eating and weight loss.

- The FastDiet demands that we think about not just *what* we eat, but *when* we eat it.

- There are no complicated rules to follow; the strategy is flexible, comprehensible, and user-friendly.

- There is no daily slog of calorie control—none of the boredom, frustration, or serial deprivation that characterizes conventional diet plans.

- Yes, it involves fasting, but not as you know it; you won't "starve" on any given day.

- You will still enjoy the foods you love—most of the time.

- Once the weight is off, sticking to the basic program will mean that it stays off.

- Weight loss is only one benefit of the FastDiet. The real dividend is the potential long-term health gains—cutting your risk of a range of diseases, including diabetes, heart disease, and cancer.

- You will soon come to understand that it is not a diet. It is much more than that: it is a sustainable strategy for a healthy, long life.

Now you'll want to understand exactly how we can make these dramatic assertions. In the next chapter, Michael explains the science that makes the FastDiet tick.

CHAPTER ONE

The Science of Fasting

OR MOST ANIMALS OUT IN THE WILD, PERIODS OF feast or famine are the norm. Our remote ancestors did not often eat four or five times a day. Instead they would kill, gorge, lie around, and then have to go for long periods of time without having anything to eat. Our bodies and our genes were forged in an environment of scarcity, punctuated by the occasional massive blowout.

These days, of course, things are very different. We eat all the time. Fasting—the voluntary abstaining from eating food—is seen as a rather eccentric, not to mention unhealthy, thing to do. Most of us expect to eat at least three meals a day and have substantial snacks in between. In between the meals and the snacks, we also graze: a milky cappuccino here, the odd cookie there, or maybe a smoothie because it's "healthier."

Once upon a time, parents told their children, "Don't eat between meals." Those times are long gone. Recent research in the United States, which compared the eating habits of 28,000 children and 36,000 adults over the last thirty years, found that the amount of time between what the researchers coyly described as "eating occasions" has fallen by an average of an hour. In other words, over the last few decades the amount of time we spend "not eating" has dropped dramatically.[1] In the 1970s, adults would go about four and a half hours without eating, while children would be expected to last about four hours between meals. Now it's down to three and a half hours for adults and three hours for children, and that doesn't include all the drinks and nibbles.

The idea that eating little and often is a "good thing" has been driven partly by snack manufacturers and faddish diet books, but it has also had support from the medical establishment. Their argument is that it is better to eat lots of small meals because that way we are less likely to get hungry and gorge on high-fat junk. I can appreciate the argument, and there have been some studies that suggest there are health benefits to eating small meals regularly, as long as you don't simply end up eating more. Unfortunately, in the real world that's exactly what happens.

In the study I quoted above, the authors found that compared to thirty years ago, we not only eat around 180 calories a day more in snacks—much of it in the form of milky drinks, smoothies, carbonated beverages—but we also eat more when it comes to our regular meals, up by an average of 120 calories a day. In other words, snacking doesn't seem to mean that we eat less at mealtimes; it just whets the appetite.

Eating throughout the day is now so normal, so much the expected thing to do, that it is almost shocking to suggest there is value in doing the absolute opposite. When I first started fasting, I discovered some unexpected things about myself, my beliefs, and my attitudes to food.

- I discovered that I often eat when I don't need to. I do it because the food is there, because I am afraid that I will get hungry later or simply from habit.

- I assumed that when you get hungry, it builds and builds until it becomes intolerable, and so you bury your face in a vat of ice cream. I found instead that hunger passes, and once you have been really hungry, you no longer fear it.

- I thought that fasting would make me distractible, unable to concentrate. What I've discovered is that it sharpens my senses and my brain.

I thought that fasting would make me distractible, unable to concentrate. What I've discovered is that it sharpens my senses and my brain.

- I wondered if I would feel faint for much of the time. It turns out the body is incredibly adaptable, and many athletes I've spoken to advocate training while fasting.

- I feared it would be incredibly hard to do. It isn't.

Why I Got Started

Although most of the great religions advocate fasting (the Sikhs are an exception, although they do allow fasting for medical reasons), I have always assumed that this was principally a way of testing yourself and your faith. I could see potential spiritual benefits, but I was deeply skeptical about the physical benefits.

I have also had a number of body-conscious friends who, down the years, have tried to get me to fast, but I could never accept their explanation that the reason for doing so was "to rest the liver" or "to remove the toxins." Neither explanation made any sense to a medically trained skeptic like me. I remember one friend telling me that after a couple of weeks of fasting, his urine had turned black, proof that the toxins were leaving. I saw it as proof that he was an ignorant hippie and that whatever was going on inside his body as a result of fasting was extremely damaging.

As I wrote in the introduction, what convinced me to try fasting was a combination of my own personal circumstances—in my midfifties, with high blood sugar, slightly overweight—and the emerging scientific evidence, which I list below.

That Which Does Not Kill Us Makes Us Stronger

There were a number of researchers who inspired me in different ways, but one who stands out is Dr. Mark Mattson of the National Institute on Aging in Bethesda, Maryland. A couple of years ago he wrote an article with Edward Calabrese in *NewScientist* magazine. Entitled "When a little poison is good for you,"[2] it really made me sit up and think.

"A little poison is good for you" is a colorful way of describing the theory of hormesis—the idea that when a human, or indeed any other creature, is exposed to a stress or toxin, it can toughen them up. Hormesis is not just a variant of "join the army and it will make a man of you"; it is now a well-accepted biological explanation of how things operate at the cellular level.

Take, for example, something as simple as exercise. When you run or pump iron, what you are actually doing is damaging your muscles, causing small tears and rips. If you don't completely overdo it, then your body responds by doing repairs, making the muscles stronger in the process.

Vegetables are another example. We all know that we should eat lots of fruits and vegetables because they are chock-full of antioxidants—and antioxidants are great because they mop up the dangerous free radicals that roam our bodies doing harm.

The trouble with this widely accepted explanation of how fruit and vegetables "work" is that it is almost certainly wrong, or at least incomplete. The levels of antioxidants in fruits and vegetables are far too low to have the profound effects they clearly do. In addition, the attempts to extract antioxidants from plants and then give them to us in a concentrated form as a health-inducing supplement have been unconvincing when tested in long-term trials. Beta carotene, when you get it in the form of a carrot, is undoubtedly good for you. When beta carotene was taken out of the carrot and given as a supplement to patients with cancer, it actually seemed to make them worse.

A clue to a completely different way that vegetables may be working comes from thinking about them through the prism of hormesis.

Consider this apparent paradox: Bitterness is often associated in the wild with poison, something to be avoided. Plants produce a huge range of so-called phytochemicals, and some of them act as natural pesticides to keep mammals like us from eating them. The fact that they taste bitter is a clear warning signal: "keep away." So there are good evolutionary reasons why we should dislike and avoid bitter-tasting foods. Yet some of the vegetables that are particularly good for us, such as cabbage, cauliflower, broccoli, and other members of the genus *Brassica*, are so bitter that even as adults many of us struggle to love them.

The resolution to this paradox is that these vegetables taste bitter because they contain chemicals that are potentially poisonous. The reason they don't harm us is that these chemicals exist in vegetables at low doses that are not toxic. Instead they activate stress responses and switch on genes that protect and repair.

Fasting and Hormesis

Once you start looking at the world in this way, you realize that many activities we initially find stressful—eating bitter vegetables, going for a run, intermittent fasting—are far from harmful. The challenge itself seems to be part of the benefit. The fact that prolonged starvation is clearly very bad for you does not imply that short periods of intermittent fasting must be a little bit bad for you. In fact the reverse is true.

This point was vividly made to me by Dr. Valter Longo, director of the University of Southern California's Longevity Institute. His research is mainly into the study of why we age, particularly concerning approaches that reduce the risk of developing age-related diseases such as cancer and diabetes.

I went to see Valter, not just because he is a world expert, but also because he had kindly agreed to act as my fasting mentor and buddy, to help inspire and guide me through my first experience of fasting.

Valter has not only been studying fasting for many years, he is also a keen adherent of it. He lives by his research and thrives on the sort of low-protein, high-vegetable diet that his grandparents enjoy in southern Italy. Perhaps not coincidentally, his grandparents live in a part of Italy that has an extraordinarily high concentration of long-lived people.

As well as following a fairly strict diet, Valter skips lunch to keep his weight down. Beyond this, once every six months or so he does a prolonged fast that lasts several days. Tall, slim, energetic, and Italian, he is an inspiring poster boy for would-be fasters.

The main reason he is so enthusiastic about fasting is that his research, and that of others, has demonstrated the extraordinary range of measurable health benefits you get from doing it. Going without food for even quite short periods of time switches on a number of so-called repair genes, which, as he explained, can confer long-term benefits. "There is a lot of initial evidence to suggest that temporary periodic fasting can induce long-lasting changes that can be beneficial against aging and diseases," he told me. "You take a person, you fast them, after twenty-four hours everything is revolutionized. And even if you took a cocktail of drugs, very potent drugs, you will never even get close to what fasting does. The beauty of fasting is that it's all coordinated."

There is a lot of initial evidence to suggest that temporary periodic fasting can induce long-lasting changes that can be beneficial against aging and diseases.

Fasting and Longevity

Most of the early long-term studies on the benefits of fasting were done on rodents. They gave us important insights into the molecular mechanisms that underpin fasting.

In one early study from 1945, rats were fasted for either one day in four, one day in three, or one day in two. The researchers found that the fasted rats lived longer than a control group, and that the more they fasted, the longer they lived. They also found that unlike perpetually calorie-restricted rats, the fasted rats were not physically stunted.[3]

Since then, numerous studies have confirmed, at least in rodents, the value of fasting. But why does fasting help? What is the mechanism?

Valter has access to his own supply of genetically engineered mice known as dwarf or Laron mice, which he was keen to show me. These mice, though small, hold the record for longevity extension in a mammal. In other words, they live for an astonishingly long time.

The average mouse doesn't live that long, perhaps two years. Laron mice live nearly twice that, many for almost four years when they are also calorie restricted. In a human, that would be the equivalent of reaching almost 170.

The fascinating thing about Laron mice is not just how long they live, but that they stay healthy for most of their very long lives. They simply don't seem to be prone to diabetes or cancer, and when they die, more often than not it is of natural causes. Valter told me that during an autopsy, it is often impossible to find a cause of death. The mice just seem to drop dead.

The reason these mice are so small and so long-lived is that they are genetically engineered so that their bodies do not respond to a hormone called IGF-1, insulin-like growth factor 1. IGF-1, as its name implies, has growth-promoting effects on almost every cell in the body. In other words, it keeps your cells constantly active. You need adequate levels of IGF-1 and other growth factors when you are young and growing, but high levels later in life appear to lead to accelerated aging and cancer. As Valter puts it, it's like driving along with your foot flat down on the accelerator pedal, pushing the car to continue to perform all the time. "Imagine, instead of occasionally taking your car to the garage and changing parts and pieces, you simply kept on driving it and driving it and driving it. Well, the car, of course, is going to break down."

Valter's work is focused on trying to figure out how you can go on driving as much as possible, and as fast as possible, while enjoying life. He thinks the answer is periodic fasting. Because one of the ways fasting works is by making your body reduce the amount of IGF-1 it produces.

The evidence that IGF-1 plays a key role in many of the diseases of aging comes not just from engineered rodents like the Laron mice, but also from humans. For the last seven years, Valter has been studying villagers in Ecuador with a genetic defect called Laron syndrome or Laron-type dwarfism. This is an extremely rare condition that affects fewer than 350 people in the entire world. People with Laron syndrome have a mutation in their growth hormone receptor (GHR) and very low levels of IGF-1. The genetically engineered Laron mice have a similar type of GHR mutation.

The villagers with Laron syndrome are normally quite short; many are less than four feet tall. The thing that is most surprising about them, however, is that like the Laron mice, they simply don't seem to develop common diseases like diabetes and cancer. In fact, Valter says that though they have been studied for many years, he has not come across a single case of someone with Laron dying of cancer. Yet their relatives, who live in the same household but who don't have Laron syndrome, do get cancer.

Disappointingly for anyone hoping that IGF-1 will provide the secrets of immortality, people with Laron syndrome—unlike the mice—are not that exceptionally long-lived. They certainly lead long lives, but not extremely long lives. Valter thinks one reason for this may be that they tend to enjoy life rather than worry about their lifestyle. "They smoke, eat a high-calorie diet, and then they look at me and they say, 'Oh it doesn't matter, I'm immune.' "

Valter thinks they prefer the idea of living as they want and dying at age 85, rather than living more carefully and perhaps going beyond 100. He would like to persuade some of them to take on a healthier lifestyle and see what happens, but knows he wouldn't live long enough to see the outcome.

Fasting and Repair Genes

As well as reducing circulating levels of IGF-1, fasting also appears to switch on a number of repair genes. The reason this happens is not fully understood, but the evolutionary argument goes something like this: As long as we have plenty of food, our bodies are mainly interested in growing, having sex, and reproducing. Nature has no long-term plans for us; she does not invest in our old age. Once we've reproduced, we become disposable. So what happens if you decide to fast? Well, the body's initial reaction is one of shock. Signals go to the brain reminding you that you are hungry, urging you to go out and find something to eat. But you resist. The body now decides that the reason you are not eating as much and as frequently as you usually do must be because you are now in a famine situation. In the past this would have been quite normal.

In a famine situation, there is no point in expending energy on growth or sex. Instead, the wisest thing the body can do is to spend its precious store of energy on repair, trying to keep you in reasonable shape until the good times return once more. The result is that as well as removing its foot from the accelerator, your body takes itself along to the cellular equivalent of a garage. There, all the little gene mechanics are ordered to start doing some of the urgent maintenance tasks that have been put off till now.

One of the things that calorie restriction does, for example, is to switch on a process called autophagy.[4] Autophagy, meaning "self-eat," is a process by which the body breaks down and recycles old and tired cells. Just as with a car, it is important to get rid of damaged or aging parts if you are going to keep things in good working order.

Valter thinks that the majority of people with a BMI over 25 would benefit from fasting, but he also thinks that if you plan to do it for more than a day, it should be done in a proper center. As he puts it, "A prolonged fast is an extreme intervention. If it's done well, it can be very powerful in your favor. If it's done improperly, it can be very powerful against you." With a prolonged fast lasting several days, you also have a drop in blood pressure and some fairly profound metabolic reprogramming. Some people faint. It's not common, but it happens.

One of Valter's areas of research is into the effects of fasting on cancer (see more on page 47), and this seems to be optimized by prolonged rather than intermittent fasting. As he pointed out, the first time you try fasting for a few days, it can be a bit of a struggle. "Our bodies are used to high levels of glucose and high levels of insulin, so it takes time to adapt. But then eventually it's not that hard."

I wasn't keen to hear "eventually," but by then I knew I would have to give it a go. It was a challenge, and one I thought I could win. Brain against stomach. No contest.

Experiencing a Four-Day Fast

I don't think it is either necessary or particularly desirable to do a prolonged fast before embarking on the FastDiet. While there are few known risks involved in fasting for less than twenty-four hours, as I explained above, there are risks attached to prolonged fasts. I decided to start with a four-day fast because I knew I was in safe hands. I had also had my IGF-1 levels measured just before I met Valter, and they were high. Not super high, as he kindly put it, but at the top end of the range (see my data on page 58).

High levels of IGF-1 are associated with a range of cancers, amongst them prostate cancer, which troubled my father. Would a four-day fast change anything?

I had been warned that the first few days might be tough, but after that I would start feeling the effects of a rush of what Valter termed well-being chemicals. Even better, the next time I fasted would be easier, because my body and brain would have a memory of it and understand what it was I was going through.

Having decided that I would try an extended fast, my next decision was how harsh to make it. A number of different countries have a tradition of fasting. The Russians seem to prefer it tough. For them, a fast consists of nothing but water, cold showers, and exercise. The Germans, on the other hand, prefer their fasts to be considerably gentler. Go to a fasting clinic in Germany and you will probably be fed around 200 calories a day in comfortable surroundings.

I wanted to see results, so I went for a British compromise. I would eat 25 calories a day, no cold showers, and just try working normally.

So on a warm Monday evening I enjoyed my last meal, an extremely filling dinner of steak, fries, and salad, washed down with beer. I felt a certain trepidation as I realized that for the next four days I would be drinking nothing but water, sugarless black tea, and coffee, and eating one measly cup of low-calorie soup a day.

Despite what I'd been told and read, before I began my fast I secretly feared that hunger would grow and grow, gnawing away inside me until I finally gave in and ran amok in a cake shop. The first twenty-four hours were quite tough, just as Valter had predicted, but as he also predicted, things got better, not worse. Yes, there were hunger pangs, sometimes quite distracting, but if I kept busy they went away.

During the first twenty-four hours of a fast there are some very profound changes going on inside the body. Within a few hours, glucose circulating in the blood is consumed. If that's not being replaced by food, then the body turns to glycogen, a stable form of glucose that is stored in the muscles and liver.

Only when that's gone does it really switch on fat burning. What actually happens is that fatty acids are broken down in the liver, resulting in the production of something called ketone bodies. These ketone bodies are now used by the brain instead of glucose as a source of energy.

> During the first twenty-four hours of a fast there are some very profound changes going on inside the body.

The first two days of a fast can be uncomfortable because your body and brain are having to cope with the switch from using glucose and glycogen as a fuel to using ketone bodies. The body is not used to them, so you can get headaches, though I didn't. You may find it hard to sleep. I didn't. The biggest problem I had with fasting is hard to put into words; it was sometimes just feeling "uncomfortable." I can't really describe it more accurately than that. I didn't feel faint, I just felt out of place.

I did, occasionally, feel hungry, but most of the time I was surprisingly cheerful. By day three the feel-good hormones had come to my rescue.

By Friday, day four, I was almost disappointed that it was ending. Almost. Despite Valter's warning that it would be unwise to gorge immediately upon breaking a fast, I got myself a plate of bacon and eggs and settled down to eat. After a few mouthfuls I was full. I really didn't need any more and in fact skipped lunch.

That afternoon I had myself tested again and discovered I had lost just under three pounds of body weight, a significant portion of which was fat. I was also happy to see that my blood glucose levels had fallen substantially and that my IGF-1 levels, which had been right at the top end of the recommended range, had gone right down. In fact, they had almost halved. This was all good news. I had lost some fat, my blood results were looking good, and I had learned that I can control my hunger. Valter was extremely pleased with these changes, particularly the fall in IGF-1, which he said would significantly reduce my risk of cancer. But he also warned me that if I went back to my old lifestyle, these changes would not be permanent.

Valter's research points toward the fact that high levels of protein, the amounts found in a typical Western diet, help keep IGF-1 levels high. I knew that there is protein in foods like meat and fish, but I was surprised there is so much in milk. I used to like drinking a skinny latte most mornings. I had the illusion that because it is made of skim milk, it is healthy. Unfortunately, though low in fat, a large latte comes in at around 11 grams of protein. The recommendation is that you stick to government guidelines, which can be found at websites like http://www.cdc.gov/nutrition /everyone/basics/protein.html. Recommended levels vary according to age and gender. They are around 46 grams of protein for women between 19 and 75, and 55 grams of protein for men between 19 and 75. I realized that the lattes would have to go.

Fasting and Weight Loss

One way to lose weight would be to go on a prolonged fast. I did the four-day fast, as described above, mainly because I was curious. I would not recommend it as a weight-loss regimen because it is completely unsustainable. Unless they combine it with vigorous exercise, people who go on prolonged fasts lose muscle as well as fat. Then, when they stop (as they must eventually do), the risk is they will pile the weight right back on.

Fortunately, less drastic, intermittent fasting, the subject of this book, leads to steady weight loss, which seems to be both sustainable and without muscle loss.

ADF, Alternate-Day Fasting

One of the most extensively studied forms of short-term fasting is alternate-day fasting. As its name implies, it means you eat no food, or relatively little food, every other day. One of the few researchers to have done human studies in this area is Dr. Krista Varady of the University of Illinois at Chicago. This plan had also been called alternate-day modified fasting (ADMF).

Krista is slim, charming, and very amusing. We met in an old-fashioned American diner, where I guiltily ate a burger and fries while Krista told me about one of the recent studies she has been doing with human volunteers.[5] On Krista's fasting days, men are allowed around 600 calories a day; women, 500 calories a day. On her regimen you eat all your calories in one go, normally as lunch. On your feed days you are allowed to eat broadly what you want.

What surprised Krista is that, although they are allowed to, people don't go crazy on their feed days. "I thought when I started running these trials that people would eat 175 percent the next day; they'd just fully compensate and wouldn't lose any weight. But most people eat around 110 percent, just slightly over what they usually eat. I haven't measured it yet, but I think it involves stomach size, how far that can expand out. Because eating almost twice the amount of food that you normally eat is actually pretty difficult. You can do it over time; people that are obese, their stomachs get bigger to accommodate, you know, 5,000 calories a day. But just to do it right off is actually pretty difficult."

In her earlier studies, the subjects were asked to stick to a low-fat diet, but what Krista wanted to know was whether ADF would also work if her subjects were allowed to eat a typical American high-fat diet. So she asked thirty-three obese volunteers, most of them women, to go on ADF for eight weeks. Before starting, the volunteers were divided into two groups. One group was put on a low-fat diet, eating low-fat cheeses and dairy, very lean meats, and a lot of fruit and vegetables. The other group was allowed to eat high-fat lasagna, pizza, the sort of diet a typical American might consume. Americans consume somewhere between 35 and 45 percent fat in their diet.

As Krista explained, the results were unexpected. The researchers and the volunteers had assumed that the people on the low-fat diet would lose more weight than those on the high-fat diet. But if anything, it was the other way around. The volunteers on the high-fat diet lost an average of 12.32 pounds, while those on the low-fat diet lost 9.24 pounds. They both lost about 2.75 inches around their waists.

Krista thinks that the main reason this happened was compliance. The volunteers randomized to the high-fat diet were more likely to stick to it than those on the low-fat diet simply because they found it a lot more palatable. And it wasn't just weight loss. Both groups saw impressive drops in LDL cholesterol (the bad cholesterol) and in blood pressure.

This meant that they had reduced their risk of cardiovascular disease, of having a heart attack or stroke.

Krista doesn't want to encourage people to binge on rubbish. She would much rather that people on ADF increase their intake of fruit and vegetables. The trouble is, as she pointed out rather exasperatedly, doctors have been encouraging people to embrace a healthy lifestyle for decades, and not enough of us are doing it. She thinks dietitians should take into account what people actually do rather than what we would like them to do.

One other significant benefit to intermittent fasting is that you don't seem to lose muscle, which you would on a normal calorie-restricted regimen. Krista herself is not sure why that is and wants to do further research.

The Two-Day Fast

One of the problems with ADF, which is why I am not so keen on it, is that you have to do it every other day. In my experience this can be socially inconvenient as well as emotionally demanding. There is no pattern to your week and other people, friends, and family, find it hard to keep track of when your fast and feed days are.

Unlike Krista's subjects, I was not particularly overweight to start with, so I also worried about losing too much weight too rapidly. That is why, having tried ADF for a short while, I decided to cut back to fasting two days a week. But more on that later in this chapter.

I now have my own experience of this to fall back on (see page 52), together with the experiences of hundreds of others who have written to me over the last few months. But what trials have been done on two-day fasts in humans?

Dr. Michelle Harvie, a dietitian based at the Genesis Breast Cancer Prevention Centre at the Wythenshawe Hospital in Manchester, England, has done a number of studies assessing the effects of a two-day fast on female volunteers. In a recent study, she divided 115 women into three groups. One group was asked to stick to a 1,500-calorie Mediterranean diet, and was also encouraged to avoid high-fat foods and alcohol.[6] Another group was asked to eat normally on five days a week, but to eat a 650-calorie, low-carbohydrate diet on the other two days. A final group was asked to avoid carbohydrates for two days a week, but was otherwise not calorie restricted.

After three months, the women on the two-day diets had lost an average of 8.80 pounds, which was almost twice as much as the full-time dieters, who had lost an average of just 5.28 pounds. Insulin resistance had also improved significantly in the two-day diet groups (see more on insulin on page 43).

The focus of Michelle's work is trying to reduce breast cancer risk through dietary interventions. Being obese and having high levels of insulin resistance are both risk factors. On the Genesis website (www.genesisuk.org), she points out that they have been studying intermittent fasting at the Genesis Breast Cancer Prevention Centre, University Hospital of South Manchester NHS Foundation Trust, for over six years and that their research has shown that cutting down on your calories for two days a week gives the same benefits, possibly more, than by going on a normal calorie-restricted diet. "To date, our research has concluded that intermittent diets appear to be a safe, viable, alternative approach to weight loss and maintaining a lower weight, in comparison to daily dieting."

> To date, our research has concluded that intermittent diets appear to be a safe, viable, alternative approach to weight loss and maintaining a lower weight, in comparison to daily dieting.

Is It Just Calories?

If you eat 500 or 600 calories two days a week and don't significantly overcompensate during the rest of the week, then you will lose weight in a steady fashion.

But is there any evidence that intermittent fasting does more than that? I recently came across one particularly fascinating study suggesting that when you eat can be almost as important as what you eat.

In this study, scientists from the Salk Institute for Biological Studies took two groups of mice and fed them a high-fat diet.[7] All the mice got exactly the same amount of food to eat, the only difference being that the mice in one group were allowed to eat whenever they wanted, nibbling away when they were in the mood, rather like we do, while the mice in the other group had to eat their food within an eight-hour time period. This meant that there were sixteen hours of the day in which they were, involuntarily, fasting.

After 100 days, there were some truly dramatic differences between the two groups of mice. The mice who nibbled away at their fatty food had developed high cholesterol and high blood glucose, and had liver damage. The mice that had been forced to fast for sixteen hours a day put on far less weight (28 percent less) and suffered much less liver damage, despite having eaten exactly the same amount and quality of food. They also had lower levels of chronic inflammation, which suggests they had reduced risk of a number of diseases including heart disease, cancer, stroke, and Alzheimer's.

The Salk researchers' explanation for this is that all the time you are eating, your insulin levels are elevated and your body is stuck in fat-storing mode (see the discussion of insulin on page 43). Only after a few hours of fasting is your body able to turn off the fat-storing and turn on the fat-burning mechanisms. So if you are a mouse and you are continually nibbling, your body will just continue making and storing fat, resulting in obesity and liver damage.

By now, I hope you are as convinced as I am that fasting offers multiple health benefits, as well as helping to achieve weight loss. I had been aware of some of these claims before I got really interested in fasting and, though initially skeptical, I was converted by the sheer weight of evidence.

But there was one area of study that was a complete surprise: research showing how fasting can improve mood and protect the brain from dementia and cognitive decline. This, for me, was something completely new, unexpected, and hugely exciting.

> But there was one area of study that was a complete surprise: research showing how fasting can improve mood and protect the brain from dementia and cognitive decline.

Fasting and the Brain

The brain, as Woody Allen once said, is my second favorite organ. I might even put it first, as without it nothing else would function. The brain, around three pounds of pinkish-grayish gunk with the consistency of tapioca, has been described as the most complex object in the known universe. It allows us to build, write poetry, dominate the planet, and even understand ourselves, something no other creature has succeeded in doing.

It is also an extremely efficient energy-saving machine, doing all that complicated thinking and making sure our bodies are functioning properly while using the same amount of energy as a 25-watt light bulb. The fact that our brains are normally so flexible and adaptable makes it even more tragic when they go wrong. I am aware that as I get older my memory has become more fallible. I've compensated by using a range of memory tricks I've picked up over the years, but even so, I find myself occasionally struggling to remember names and dates. Far worse than this, however, is the fear that one day I may lose my mind entirely, perhaps developing some form of dementia. Obviously I want to preserve my brain in as good a shape as possible and for as long as possible. Fortunately fasting seems to offer significant protection.

The man I went to discuss my brain with was Mark Mattson.

Mark, who is Chief of the Laboratory of Neurosciences at the National Institute on Aging, is one of the most revered scientists in his field, the study of the aging brain. I find his work genuinely inspiring—suggesting, as it does, that fasting can help combat diseases like Alzheimer's, dementia, and memory loss.

Although I could have taken a taxi to his office, I chose to walk. I'm a fan of walking. It not only burns calories, it also improves the mood, and it may also help you retain your memory. Normally, as we get older, our brain shrinks, but one study found that in regular walkers the hippocampus, the area of the brain essential for memory, actually expanded.[8] Regular walkers have brains that in MRI scans look, on average, two years younger than the brains of those who are sedentary.

Mark, who studies Alzheimer's, lost his own father to dementia. He told me that although it didn't directly motivate him to go into this particular line of research—when he started his work on Alzheimer's disease, his father had not yet been diagnosed—it did give him insight into the condition.

Alzheimer's affects around 26 million people worldwide, and the problem will grow as the population ages. New approaches are desperately needed because the tragedy of Alzheimer's disease and other forms of dementia is that once you're diagnosed, it may be possible to delay, but not prevent, the inevitable deterioration. You are likely to get progressively worse to the point where you need constant care for many years. By the end, you may not even recognize the faces of those you once loved.

So what can fasting do?

Just as Valter Longo had, Mark took me off to see some mice. Like Valter's mice, these were genetically engineered, but Mark's mice had been modified to make them more vulnerable to Alzheimer's. The mice I saw were in a maze that they had to navigate in order to find food. Some of the mice performed this task with relative ease; others got disorientated and confused. This task and others like it are designed to reveal signs that the mice are developing memory problems; a mouse that is struggling will quickly forget which arm of the maze it has already traveled down.

If put on a normal diet, the genetically engineered Alzheimer's mice will quickly develop dementia. By the time they are a year old, the equivalent of middle age in humans, they normally have obvious learning and memory problems. The animals put on an intermittent fast, something Mark prefers to call "intermittent energy restriction," often go for up to twenty months without any detectable signs of dementia.[9] They only really start deteriorating toward the end of their lives. That's the equivalent in a human of the difference between developing signs of Alzheimer's at the age of 50 and the age of 80. I know which I would prefer.

Disturbingly, when these mice are put on a typical junk-food diet, they go downhill much earlier than even normally fed mice. "We put mice on a high-fat and high-fructose diet," Mark said, "and that has a dramatic effect; the animals have an earlier onset of the learning and memory problems, more accumulation of amyloid, and more problems with finding their way in a maze test."

In other words, junk food makes these mice fat and stupid.

One of the key changes that occurs in the brains of Mark's fasting mice is increased production of a protein called brain-derived neurotrophic factor. BDNF has been shown to stimulate stem cells to turn into new nerve cells in the hippocampus. As I mentioned earlier, this is a part of the brain that is essential for normal learning and memory.

But why should the hippocampus grow in response to fasting? Mark points out that from an evolutionary perspective it makes sense. After all, the times when you need to be smart and on the ball are when there's not a lot of food lying around. "If an animal is in an area where there's limited food resources, it's important that they are able to remember where food is, remember where hazards are, predators and so on. We think that people in the past who were able to respond to hunger with increased cognitive ability had a survival advantage."

We don't know for sure if humans grow new brain cells in response to fasting; to be absolutely certain, researchers would need to put volunteers on an intermittent fast and then kill them, take their brains out, and look for signs of new neural growth. It seems unlikely that many would volunteer for such a project. But researchers are doing a study in which volunteers fast and then MRI scans are used to see if the size of their hippocampi has changed over time.

As I mentioned above, these techniques have been used in humans to show that regular exercise, such as walking, increases the size of the hippocampus. Hopefully, similar studies will show that two days a week of intermittent fasting are good for learning and memory. On a purely anecdotal level, and using a sample size of one, it seems to work. Before starting the FastDiet, I did a sophisticated memory test online. Two months in I repeated the test, and my performance had, indeed, improved. If you are interested in doing something similar, then I suggest you go to cognitivefun.net/test/2.

Fasting and Mood

One of the things that Valter Longo and others told me before I began my four-day fast was that it would be tough initially, but that after a while I would start to feel more cheerful, which was indeed what happened. Similarly, I was surprised to discover how positive I have felt while doing intermittent fasting. I expected to feel tired and crabby on my fasting days, but that didn't happen at all. So is this improved mood simply a psychological effect—that people who do intermittent fasting and lose weight feel good about themselves—or are there also chemical changes that are influencing mood?

According to Mark Mattson, one of the reasons people may find intermittent fasting relatively easy to do is because of its effects on brain-derived neurotrophic factor. BDNF not only seems to protect the brain against the ravages of dementia and age-related mental decline, but it may also improve your mood.

There have been a number of studies going back many years that suggest rising levels of BDNF have an antidepressant effect; at least they do in rodents. In one study, researchers injected BDNF directly into the brains of rats and found this had similar effects to repeated use of a standard antidepressant.[10] Another paper found that electroshock therapy, which is known to be effective in severe depression in human patients, seems to work, at least in part, because it stimulates the production of higher levels of BDNF.[11]

Mark Mattson believes that within a few weeks of starting a two-day-a-week fasting regimen, BDNF levels will start to rise, suppressing anxiety and elevating mood. He doesn't currently have the human data to fully support this claim, but he is doing trials on volunteers in which, among other things, his team is collecting regular samples of cerebrospinal fluid (the liquid that bathes the brain and spinal cord) in order to measure the changes that occur during intermittent fasts. This is not a trial for the faint-hearted, as it requires regular spinal taps, but as Mark pointed out to me, many of his volunteers are already undergoing early signs of cognitive change, so they are extremely motivated.

Mark is keen to study and promote the benefits of intermittent fasting, as he is genuinely worried about the likely effects of the current obesity epidemic on our brains and our society. He also thinks that if you are considering intermittent fasting, you should get going sooner rather than later: "The age-related cognitive decline in Alzheimer's disease, the events that are occurring in the brain at the level of the nerve cells and the molecules in the nerve cells, those changes are occurring very early, probably decades before the subject starts to have learning and memory problems. That's why it's critical to start dietary regimens early on, when people are young or middle-aged, so that they can slow down the development of these processes in the brain and live to be ninety with their brain functioning perfectly well."

Like Mark, I'm convinced the human brain benefits from short periods abstaining from food. This is an exciting and fast-emerging area of research that many will watch with great interest. Beyond the brain, though, intermittent fasting also has measurable, beneficial effects on other areas in the body—on the heart, on blood profile, on cancer risk. And that's where we'll turn now.

Beyond the brain, though, intermittent fasting also has measurable, beneficial effects on other areas in the body—on the heart, on blood profile, on cancer risk.

Fasting and Your Biochemistry

One of the main reasons I decided to try fasting was that I had tests suggesting I was heading for serious problems with my cardiovascular system. Nothing had happened yet, but the warning signs were flashing amber. The tests showed that my blood levels of LDL (low-density lipoprotein, the "bad" cholesterol) were disturbingly high, as were the levels of my fasting glucose.

To measure fasting glucose, you have to fast overnight, then give a sample of blood. The normal, desirable range is 3.9 to 5.8 mmol/l. Mine was 7.3 mmol/l. Not yet diabetic, but dangerously high. There are many reasons that you should do all you can to avoid becoming a diabetic, not the least the fact that it dramatically increases your risk of having a heart attack or stroke.

Fasting glucose is an important thing to measure because it is an indicator that all may not be well with your insulin levels.

Insulin: The Fat-Making Hormone

When we eat food, particularly foods rich in carbohydrates, our blood glucose levels rise and the pancreas, an organ tucked away below the ribs next to the left kidney, starts to churn out insulin. Glucose is the main fuel that our cells use for energy, but the body does not like having high levels of it circulating in the blood. The job of insulin, a hormone, is to regulate blood glucose levels, ensuring that they are neither too high nor too low. It normally does this with great precision. The problem comes when the pancreas gets overloaded.

Insulin is a sugar controller; it aids the extraction of glucose from blood and then stores it in places like your liver or muscles in a stable form called glycogen, to be used when and if it is needed. What is less commonly known is that insulin is also a fat controller. It inhibits something called lipolysis, the breakdown of stored body fat. At the same time, it forces fat cells to take up and store fat from your blood. Insulin makes you fat. High levels lead to increased fat storage, low levels to fat depletion.

The trouble with constantly eating lots of sugary, carbohydrate-rich foods and drinks, as we increasingly do, is that this requires the release of more and more insulin to deal with the glucose surge. Up to a point, your pancreas will cope by simply pumping out ever-larger quantities of insulin. This leads to greater fat deposition and also increases cancer risk. Naturally enough, this can't go on forever. If you continue to produce ever-larger quantities of insulin, your cells will eventually rebel and become resistant to its effects. It's rather like shouting at your children; you can keep escalating things, but after a certain point they will simply stop listening.

Eventually the cells stop responding to insulin; your blood glucose levels now stay permanently high, and you will find you have joined the 285 million people around the world who have type 2 diabetes, a massive and rapidly growing problem worldwide. Over the last twenty years, numbers have risen almost tenfold, and there is no obvious sign that this trend is slowing.

Diabetes is associated with an increased risk of heart attack, stroke, impotence, blindness, and amputation due to poor circulation. It is also associated with brain shrinkage and dementia. Not a pretty picture.

One way to prevent the downward spiral into diabetes is to do more exercise and eat foods that do not lead to such big spikes in blood glucose and that do not have such a dramatic effect on insulin levels. More on this later. There is also evidence that intermittent fasting will help.

Intermittent Fasting and Insulin

In a study published in 2005, eight healthy young men were asked to fast every other day, twenty hours a day, for two weeks.[12] On their fasting days they were allowed to eat until 10:00 p.m., then not eat again until 6:00 p.m. the following evening. They were also asked to eat heartily the rest of the time to make sure they did not lose any weight.

The idea behind the experiment was to test the so-called thrifty hypothesis, the idea that since we evolved at a time of feast or famine, the best way to eat is to mimic those times. At the end of the two weeks, there were no changes in the volunteers' weight or body fat composition, which is what the researchers had intended. There was, however, a big change in their insulin sensitivity. In other words, after just two weeks of intermittent fasting, the same amount of circulating insulin now had a much greater effect on the volunteers' ability to store glucose or break down fat.

The researchers wrote jubilantly that "by subjecting healthy men to cycles of feast and famine we changed their metabolic status for the better." They also added that "to our knowledge this is the first study in humans in which an increased insulin action on whole body glucose uptake and adipose tissue lipolysis has been obtained by means of intermittent fasting."

> By subjecting healthy men to cycles of feast and famine we changed their metabolic status for the better.

I don't know what impact intermittent fasting has had on my insulin sensitivity—it's a test that is hard to do and extremely expensive—but what I do know is that the effects on my blood sugar have been spectacular. Before I started intermittent fasting, my blood glucose level was 7.3 mmol/l, well above the acceptable range of 3.9 to 5.8 mmol/l. The last time I had my level measured it was 5.0 mmol/l, still a bit high but well within the normal range.

This is an incredibly impressive response. My doctor, who was preparing to put me on medication, was astonished at such a dramatic turnaround. Doctors routinely recommend a healthy diet to patients with high blood glucose, but it usually makes only a marginal difference. Intermittent fasting could have a revolutionary, game-changing effect on the nation's health.

Fasting and Cancer

My father was a lovely man but not a particularly healthy one. Overweight for much of his life, by the time he reached his sixties he had developed not only diabetes but also prostate cancer. He had an operation to remove the prostate cancer, which left him with embarrassing urinary problems. Understandably, I am not at all keen to go down that road.

My four-day fast, under Valter Longo's supervision, had shown me that it was possible to dramatically cut my IGF-1 (insulin-like growth factor 1) levels and by doing so, hopefully, my prostate cancer risk. I later discovered that by doing intermittent fasting and being a bit more careful with my protein intake, I could keep my IGF-1 down at healthy levels. The link between growth, fasting, and cancer is worth unpacking.

The cells in our bodies are constantly multiplying, replacing dead, worn out, or damaged tissue. This is fine as long as cellular growth is under control, but sometimes a cell mutates, grows uncontrollably, and turns into a cancer. Very high levels of a cellular stimulant like IGF-1 in the blood are likely to increase the chance of this happening.

When a cancer goes rogue, the normal options are surgery, chemotherapy, or radiotherapy. Surgery is used to try to remove the tumor; chemotherapy and radiotherapy are used to try to poison it. The major problem with chemotherapy and radiotherapy is that they are not selective; as well as killing tumor cells they will also kill or damage surrounding healthy cells. They are particularly likely to damage rapidly dividing cells such as hair roots, which is why hair commonly falls out following therapy.

As I mentioned above, Valter Longo has shown that when we are deprived of food for even quite short periods of time, our body responds by slowing things down, going into repair and survival mode until food is once more abundant. That is true of normal cells. But cancer cells follow their own rules. They are, almost by definition, not under control and will go on selfishly proliferating whatever the circumstances. This "selfishness" creates an opportunity. At least in theory, if you fast just before chemotherapy, you create a situation in which your normal cells are hibernating while the cancer cells are running amok and are therefore more vulnerable.

In a paper published in 2008, Valter and colleagues showed that fasting "protects normal but not cancer cells against high-dose chemotherapy,"[13] followed by another paper in which they showed that fasting increased the efficacy of chemotherapy drugs against a variety of cancers.[14] Again, as is so often the case, this was a study done in mice. But the implications of Valter's work were not missed by an eagle-eyed administrative judge named Nora Quinn, who saw a short article about it in the *Los Angeles Times*.

I met Nora in Los Angeles. She is a feisty woman with a terrific, dry sense of humor. Nora first noticed she had a problem when, one morning, she put her hand on her breast and felt a lump the size of a walnut under her skin.

After indulging, as she put it, in the fantasy that it was a cyst, she went to the doctor; it was removed and sent to a pathologist.

"The reality of your life always comes out in pathology," she told me. When the pathology report came back, it said that she had invasive breast cancer. She had a course of radiotherapy and was about to start chemotherapy when she read about Valter's work with mice.

She tried to speak to Valter, but he wouldn't advise her because, up to that point, none of the trials he had run had been done with humans. He didn't know if it was safe for someone about to undergo chemo to fast, and he certainly wasn't going to encourage people like Nora to give it a go.

Undeterred, Nora did her own research and decided to try fasting for seven and a half days, before, during, and after her first bout of chemotherapy. Having discovered how tough it can be to do even a four-day fast while fully healthy, I'm surprised she was able to go through with it, though Nora says it's not so hard and I'm just a wimp. The results were mixed.

"After the first chemo I didn't get that sick, but my hair fell out, so I thought it wasn't working." So next time she didn't fast, and she was only medium sick. "I thought, seven and a half days of fasting to avoid being medium sick, this is a really bad deal. I am so not doing that again." So when it was time for her third course of chemo, she didn't fast. That, she now feels, was a mistake. "I got sick. I don't have words for how sick I was. I was weak, felt poisoned, and I couldn't get up. I felt like I was moving through Jell-O. It was absolutely horrible."

The cells that line the gut, like hair root cells, grow rapidly because they need to be constantly replaced. Chemotherapy can kill those cells, which is one reason that it can make people feel really ill.

By the time Nora had to undergo her fourth course of chemo, she had decided to try fasting once again. This time things went much better and she made a good recovery. She is currently cancer free.

Nora is convinced she benefitted from fasting, but it's hard to be sure because she wasn't part of a proper medical trial. Valter and his colleagues at USC did, however, study what happened to her and ten other patients with cancer who had also decided to put themselves on a fast.[15] All of them reported fewer and less severe symptoms after chemotherapy, and most of them, including Nora, saw improvements in their blood results. The white cells and platelets, for example, recovered more rapidly when they had chemo while they were fasting than when they did not.

But why did Nora go rogue? Why didn't she fast under proper supervision? She says: "I decided to fast based on years of information from animal testing. I do agree that if you are going to do crazy things like I did, you should have medical supervision. But how? None of my doctors would listen to me."

Nora's self-experiment could have gone wrong, which is just one reason why such maverick behavior is not recommended. Her experience, however, and that of the other nine cancer patients, helped inspire further studies. For example, Valter and his colleagues have recently completed phase one of a clinical trial to see if fasting around the time of chemotherapy is safe—which it seems to be. The next phase is to assess whether it makes a measurable difference. At least ten other hospitals around the world are either doing or have agreed to do clinical trials. Go to our website, www.thefastdiet.co.uk, for the latest updates.

Prevention Is Better Than Cure

Fasting, either prolonged or intermittent, will reduce your IGF-1 levels and, therefore, your risk of a number of different cancers. But what other evidence is there that intermittent fasting reduces cancer risk? As I mentioned above, Dr. Michelle Harvie, at the Genesis Breast Cancer Prevention Centre, has been working in this field for some time.

One of her recent studies looked at whether intermittent fasting can reduce a woman's risk of breast cancer.[16] In this study, she divided 107 female volunteers into two groups. One group was asked to eat a healthy Mediterranean diet but was

> Fasting, either prolonged or intermittent, will reduce your IGF-1 levels and, therefore, your risk of a number of different cancers.

restricted to around 1,500 calories a day. The other group was asked to consume roughly the same number of calories a week, but consumed differently. Two days a week they had to eat just 650 calories a day. After six months, those on the intermittent fast had lost more weight, an average of 12.76 to 14.30 pounds, their fasting insulin and insulin resistance had fallen further, and levels of inflammatory protein were also significantly down. All three measures suggest a reduced breast cancer risk.

Dr. Harvie also thinks that, from a cancer prevention perspective, the advantage of intermittent fasting over conventional weight loss is that it cuts the amount of sugar reaching breast cells, which may mean they divide less often and are less prone to turning cancerous.

Intermittent Fasting: My Personal Journey

As you've read, I started out by trying the four-day fast under Valter Longo's supervision. But despite the improvements in my blood biochemistry and his obvious enthusiasm, I could not imagine doing lengthy fasts on a regular basis for the rest of my life. So, what next? Well, having met Krista Varady and learned all about ADF (alternate-day fasting) I decided to give that a go.

After a short while, however, I realized that it was just too tough physically, socially, and psychologically. I need some pattern in my life and not being able to tell without a calendar and lengthy calculations whether I could meet friends for dinner on a particular night was irksome. I also found fasting every other day just a little too challenging. I realize that many of Krista's volunteers do manage to stick to it, but they are in a trial situation and highly motivated. It is undoubtedly an effective way to lose weight rapidly and to get powerful changes to your biochemistry, but it was not for me.

So I decided to try eating 600 calories, two days a week. It seemed a reasonable compromise and, more important, doable.

I tried eating all my food in one meal, as Krista does in her studies, but I discovered that if I skipped breakfast, I started to feel hungry and irritable well before lunch. So I split my food in two: a moderate breakfast, miss lunch, a light supper. And I did it twice a week. This I found extremely manageable.

After experimenting with different versions of fasting, I found the 5:2 approach to be the most effective and workable way for me to get the benefits of fasting and still retain a long-term commitment to a dietary plan. I think that a 5:2 FastDiet is a realistic synthesis of the current thinking on intermittent fasting, and the best way I know to guarantee success.

Before embarking on the diet I decided to get myself properly tested, to see what effects it would have on my body. The following are the tests I did. The blood tests results I give below (and other tests I have mentioned earlier) are in millimoles per liter, which is the way that blood tests are reported in the UK. It means the number of molecules of a substance you'll find in a liter of blood. American units and guidelines are not the same. American laboratories will give results in mg/dl, which means the weight of a substance, measured in milligrams, per 100 milliliters of blood. The two measures don't exactly translate, so I have stuck to my original figures. Your doctor should be happy to do these tests, in American units, and explain their significance.

Get on the Scale

The first and most obvious thing you will want to do is weigh yourself before embarking on this adventure. Initially, it is best to do this at the same time every day. First thing in the morning is, as I'm sure you know, when you will be at your lightest.

Body Fat

Ideally you should get a weighing machine that measures body fat percentage as well as weight, since what you really want to see is body fat levels fall. The cheaper machines are not fantastically reliable; they tend to underestimate the true figure, giving you a false sense of security. What they are quite good at doing, however, is measuring change. In other words, they might tell you when you start that you are 30 percent body fat when the true figure is closer to 33 percent. But they should be able to tell you when that number begins to fall.

Body fat is measured as a percentage of total weight. The machines you can buy do this by a system called impedance. There's a small electric current that runs through your body; the machine measures the resistance. It does its estimation based on the fact that muscle and other tissues are better conductors of electricity than fat. Women tend to have more body fat than men. A man with a body fat percentage of more than 25 percent would be considered overweight. For a woman it would be 30 percent.

The only way to get a truly accurate reading is with a machine called a DXA (formerly DEXA) scanner. It stands for "dual energy X-ray absorptiometry." It is expensive and, for most people, unnecessary.

Calculate Your BMI

Your body mass index (BMI) will tell you if you are overweight. To calculate your body mass index, go to a website such as nhlbisupport.com/bmi/. This will not only do the calculation, but also tell you what it means. One criticism of BMI is that someone who has a lot of muscle could get a high BMI score. This is not an issue for most of us, sadly.

Measure Your Stomach

BMI is useful, but it may not be the best predictor of future health. In a study of more than 45,000 women who were followed for sixteen years,[17] the waist-to-height ratio was a superior predictor of who would develop heart disease.

The reason the waist matters so much is because the worst sort of fat is visceral fat, which collects inside the abdomen. This is the worst sort of distribution because it causes inflammation and puts you at much higher risk of diabetes. You don't need fancy equipment to tell you if you have internal fat. All you need is a tape measure. Male or female, your waist should be less than half your height. Most people underestimate their waist size by about two inches because they rely on trouser size. Instead, measure your waist by putting the tape measure around your belly button. Be honest. A definition of optimism is someone who steps on the scale while holding their breath. You are fooling no one.

Blood Tests

You should be able to get standard tests during a routine visit to your doctor.

Fasting Glucose

I chose to measure my fasting glucose because it is a really important measure of fitness even if you are not at risk of diabetes, and it's a predictor of future health. Studies show that even moderately elevated levels of blood glucose are associated with increased risk of heart disease, stroke, and long-term cognitive problems. Ideally I would have had my insulin sensitivity measured, but that test is complex and expensive.

Cholesterol

They measure two types of cholesterol: LDL (low-density lipoprotein) and HDL (high-density lipoprotein). Broadly speaking, LDL carries cholesterol into the wall of your arteries while HDL carries it away. It is good to have a low-ish LDL and a high-ish HDL. One way you can express this is as a percentage of HDL to the sum of HDL plus LDL. Anything over 0.20 (20 percent) is good.

Triglycerides

These are a type of fat that is found in blood; they are one of the ways that the body stores calories. High levels are associated with increased risk of heart disease.

IGF-1

This is an expensive test and not available from every doctor. It is a measure of cell turnover and therefore of cancer risk. It may also be a marker for biological aging. I wanted to find out the effects of 5:2 fasting on my IGF-1. I had discovered that IGF-1 levels drop dramatically in response to a four-day fast, but after a month of normal eating they bounced right back to where they had been before.

My Data

These are the results of the physical measurements I took before starting the FastDiet.

	ME	RECOMMENDED
HEIGHT	5'11" (71 inches)	
WEIGHT	187 lbs.	
BODY MASS INDEX	26.4	19–25
% OF BODY FAT	28%	Less than 25% for men
WAIST SIZE	36 "	Less than half your height
NECK SIZE	17 "	Less than 16½"

I wasn't obese, but both my BMI and my body fat percentage told me that I was overweight. I knew from doing an

MRI (magnetic resonance imaging) scan that much of my fat was collected internally, wrapping itself in thick layers around my liver and kidneys, disturbing all sorts of metabolic pathways.

Clearly, the fat wasn't all inside my abdomen. Quite a bit had collected around my neck. This meant that I was snoring. Loudly. Neck size is a powerful predictor[18] of whether you will snore or not. A neck size above 16½ inches for men or 16 inches for women means you are in the danger zone.

	MY RESULTS IN MMOL/L	RECOMMENDED
DIABETES RISK		
FASTING GLUCOSE	7.3	3.9–5.8
HEART DISEASE FACTORS		
TRIGLYCERIDES	1.4	Less than 2.3
HDL CHOLESTEROL	1.8	0.9–1.5
LDL CHOLESTEROL	5.5	Up to 3.0
HEART DISEASE RISK		
HDL % OF TOTAL	23 %	20% and over
CANCER RISK		
SOMATOMEDIN-C (IGF-1)	28.6 nmol/l	11.3–30.9 nmol/l

According to these data, my fasting glucose was worryingly high. I was not yet a diabetic, but I had signs of what is called impaired glucose tolerance, or prediabetes. My LDL was far too high, but I was to some extent protected by the fact that my triglycerides were low and my HDL high. This is not a good picture, though.

My IGF-1 levels were also too high, suggesting rapid turnover of cells and increased cancer risk.

After three months on the FastDiet there were some re-markable changes, as you'll see in these charts.

	ME	RECOMMENDED
HEIGHT	5' 11" (71 inches)	
WEIGHT	168 lbs.	
BODY MASS INDEX	24	19–25
% OF BODY THAT IS FAT	21%	Less than 25% for men
WAIST SIZE	33"	Less than half your height
NECK SIZE	16"	Less than 16½"

I had lost about 19 pounds, and my BMI and body fat percentage became respectable. I had to go out and buy smaller belts and tighter trousers. I could fit into a dinner jacket I hadn't worn for ten years. I had also stopped snoring, which delighted my wife and quite possibly the neighbors. Even better, my blood indicators had improved in a spectacular fashion.

I had lost about 19 pounds, and my BMI and body fat percentage became respectable. I had to go out and buy smaller belts and tighter trousers.

	MY RESULTS IN MMOL/L	RECOMMENDED
DIABETES RISK		
FASTING GLUCOSE	5.0	3.9–5.8
HEART DISEASE FACTORS		
TRIGLYCERIDES	0.6	Less than 2.3
HDL CHOLESTEROL	2.1	0.9–1.5
LDL CHOLESTEROL	3.6	Up to 3.0
HEART DISEASE RISK		
HDL % OF TOTAL	37%	20% and over
CANCER RISK		
SOMATOMEDIN-C (IGF-1)	15.9 nmol/l	11.3–30.9 nmol/l

My wife, Clare, who is a doctor, was astonished. She regularly sees overweight patients with blood chemistry like mine had been and she said that none of the advice she gives them has had anything like the same effect.

For me, the particularly pleasing changes were in my fasting glucose levels and the huge drop in my IGF-1 levels, which matched the changes I had seen after doing a four-day fast.

Clare, however, felt I was losing weight too fast, that I should consolidate for a while. That is why I decided to go on a maintenance dose of fasting just one day a week. Unless it's the weekend, vacation, or a special occasion, I also regularly skip lunch.

What has happened is that my weight has stayed steady at 168 pounds and my blood markers remain in good shape. I do, however, think there is room for improvement and will shortly restart a two-day regimen and blog about it. If you are interested, visit our website, www.thefastdiet.co.uk.

So What Is the Best Way to Go About Intermittent Fasting?

Let's recap what we've learned. The reason for intermittent fasting—that is, briefly but severely restricting the amount of calories you consume—is that by doing so you are hoping to "fool" your body into thinking it is in a potential famine situation and that it needs to switch from go-go mode to maintenance mode.

The reason our bodies respond to fasting in this way is that we evolved at a time when feast or famine was the norm. Our bodies are designed to respond to stresses and shocks; it makes them healthier, tougher. The scientific term is hormesis—what does not kill you makes you stronger.

The benefits of fasting include

- Weight loss

- A reduction of IGF-1, which means that you are reducing your risk of a number of age-related diseases, such as cancer.

- The switching-on of countless repair genes in response to this stressor

- Giving your pancreas a rest, which will boost the effectiveness of the insulin it produces in response to elevated blood glucose. Increased insulin sensitivity will reduce your risk of obesity, diabetes, heart disease, and cognitive decline.

- An overall enhancement in your mood and sense of well-being. This may be a consequence of your brain producing increased levels of neurotrophic factor, which will hopefully make you more cheerful and in turn should make fasting more doable.

So much for the science. In the next chapter we discuss what to eat and how to go about starting life as an intermittent faster. How do you put the theory into practice?

CHAPTER TWO

The FastDiet in Practice

THERE ARE, AS WE'VE SEEN, GOOD CLINICAL REA-sons to start intermittent fasting. Some, such as its positive effect on blood markers, should be immediately apparent; others will become manifest over time—a cognitive boost, a self-repairing physiology, a greater chance of a longer life. But perhaps the most compelling argument for many is the promise of swift and sustained weight loss while still eating the foods you would eat normally, most of the time. You may view this as incidental to the plan's other forceful health benefits. Or it may be your primary objective. The fact is you will gain both: weight loss *and* better health, two sides of the same coin.

Michael's experience, as illustrated in the previous chapter, should have given you an idea of what to expect. This chapter will reveal more detail: explaining how to start, how it will feel, how to keep going, and how the central tenets of the FastDiet can slip easily into the rhythm of your everyday life. Then it's over to you.

What Does 500/600 Calories Look Like?

Cutting calories to a quarter of your usual daily intake is a significant commitment, so don't be surprised if your first fast day feels like a tough gig. As you progress, the fasts will become second nature and the initial sense of deprivation will diminish, particularly if you remain aware that tomorrow is another day—another day, in fact, when you can eat as you please.

Still, however you cut it, 500 or 600 calories is no picnic; it's not even half a picnic. A large café latte can clock in at over 300 calories, more if you insist on cream, while your usual lunchtime sandwich might easily consume your entire allowance in one huge bite. So be smart. Spend your calories wisely—the menu plans starting on page 130 will be useful—but it's also worth having a clear idea of favorite fast-day foods that work for you. Remember to embrace variety: differing textures, punchy flavors, color, and crunch. Together, these will keep your mouth entertained and stop it from frowning at the hardship of it all.

When to Fast

Animal studies, human studies, research, and experiments—as demonstrated in the previous chapter, evidence for the value of fasting is unequivocal. But what happens when you step out of the laboratory and into real life? When and what you eat during your fast is critical to the diet's success. So what's the optimal pattern?

Michael tried several different fasting regimens; the one he settled on as the most realistic and sustainable is a fast on two nonconsecutive days each week, allowing 600 calories a day, split between breakfast and dinner. This pattern has been called, for obvious reasons, a 5:2 diet—five days off, two days on, which means that the majority of your time is spent gloriously free from calorie-counting. On a fast day, he'll normally have breakfast with his family at around 7:30 a.m. and then aim to have dinner with them at 7:30 p.m., with nothing eaten in between. That way, he gets two twelve-hour periods without food in a twenty-four-hour day, and a happy family at the end of it.

The menu suggestions starting on page 130 are based on this pattern since it is, in his experience, the most straightforward and convincing intermittent fasting method.

Mimi, as she describes later in this chapter, found that a slightly different pattern works for her. Sticking to the FastDiet's central tenet, she eats 500 calories—but as two meals with a few snacks (an apple, some carrot sticks) in between, simply because the vast plain between breakfast and supper feels too great, too empty for comfort. There is evidence from trials conducted by Dr. Michelle Harvie[1] and others that this approach will help you lose weight, reduce your risk of breast cancer, and increase insulin sensitivity.

Which approach is better? At this point, given that the science of intermittent fasting is still in its infancy, we don't know. On purely theoretical grounds, a longer period without food (Michael's pattern) should produce better results than one when you eat smaller amounts more frequently. Dr. Krista Varady and her team in Chicago have yet to run a study in which people are allowed to consume their 500 or 600 calories as smaller meals throughout the day. They are planning to run this as a trial within the next year; we will update you. She expects that eating throughout the day will prevent the body going into a "fasted state." Since it is this fasted state that is so beneficial to us, eating lots of little meals is likely to significantly reduce the benefits.

Dr. Mark Mattson at the National Institute on Aging agrees that eating the 500 or 600 calories at one meal is likely to be better than eating several smaller meals over the course of the day. He thinks the longer the body goes without food, the greater the adaptive cellular stress response, which is particularly good for the brain.

Meanwhile, Dr. Valter Longo at the Longevity Institute at the University of Southern California would go further: with regard to IGF-1 reduction, he argues that it is better to do four consecutive days of fasting every few months, and to skip meals and adopt a plant-based, low-protein diet during the week to maintain an optimum weight. This, of course, is a no-no for most of us; fasting for long periods is simply too tough. In short, then, a 5:2 plan seems the pattern that offers the most scope for health benefits *and* the greatest level of tolerance. We await more trials, but until then it's our favored option for that crucial combination of weight loss and cheerful compliance.

Some people who don't feel hungry at breakfast would rather eat later in the day. That's fine. One of the key researchers in this field starts her day with a late breakfast at around 11:00 a.m. and finishes with supper at 7:00 p.m. That way, she's fasting for sixteen hours in a twenty-four-hour period, twice a week. Based on the mouse study cited on page 34, it may even be a better approach.

It is, however, only "better" if you actually do it, and a delayed breakfast may not suit some lifestyles, timetables, or bodies. So go with a timetable that suits you. Some fasters, for instance, appreciate the convenience and simplicity of a single 500- or 600-calorie meal, allowing them to ignore food entirely for most of the day. Whatever you choose, it must be your plan, your life. Do it with gusto, but be prepared to experiment within the limits set out by the plan.

What to Eat

It may seem curious to talk about what to eat when you are fasting. But the FastDiet is a modified program, allowing 500 calories for a woman and 600 for a man on any given fast day, making the regimen relatively comfortable and, above all, sustainable over the long term. So, yes, you do get to eat on a fast day. But it matters what you choose.

> The FastDiet is a modified program,
> allowing 500 calories for a woman and
> 600 for a man on any given fast day, making
> the regimen relatively comfortable and,
> above all, sustainable over the long term.

There are two general principles that should govern what you eat and what you avoid on a fast day. Your aim is to have food that makes you feel satisfied but stays firmly within the 500/600 calorie allowance—and the best options to achieve this are foods that are high in protein and foods with a low glycemic index. There have been a number of studies[2] demonstrating that individuals who eat a higher-protein diet feel fuller for longer (indeed, the main reason people lose weight on diets like Atkins is that they eat less). The trouble with really high protein diets, however, is that people tend to get bored with the food restrictions and give up. There is also evidence that high-protein diets are associated with higher levels of chronic inflammation and IGF-1, which in turn are associated with increased risk of heart disease and cancer.[3]

So the FastDiet does not recommend boycotting carbs entirely, or living permanently on a high-protein diet. However, on a fast day, the combination of proteins and foods with a low glycemic index will be helpful weapons in keeping hunger at bay.

Understanding the Glycemic Index

In earlier chapters, we discussed the importance of blood sugar and insulin. High levels of insulin brought about by high levels of blood sugar will encourage your body to store fat and increase your cancer risk. Another reason not to eat foods that make your blood sugar levels surge, particularly on your fast days, is that when your blood sugar crashes, as it inevitably will, you will start feeling very hungry indeed.

Carbohydrates have the biggest impact on blood sugar, but not all carbs are equal. As habitual dieters will know, one way to discover which carbs cause a big spike and which don't is to look at their glycemic index (GI). Each food gets a score out of 100, with a low score meaning that the particular food does not tend to cause a rapid rise in blood glucose. These are the ones you want.

The size of the sugar spike depends not just on the food itself, but also on how much of it you eat. For example, we tend to eat a lot more potatoes in one sitting than kiwi fruit. So there's also a measure called the glycemic load (GL), which is:

$$GL = \frac{GI \times grams\ of\ carbohydrate}{100}$$

This makes some pretty heroic assumptions about the amount of a particular food you are likely to eat as a portion, but at least it is a guide.

The reason GI and GL are interesting is not just because they are strongly predictive of future health (people on a low GL diet have less risk of diabetes, heart disease, and various cancers), but because there are so many surprises. Who would have imagined that eating a baked potato would have as big an impact on your blood glucose as eating a tablespoon of sugar?

Broadly speaking, a GI over 50 or a GL over 20 is not good, and the lower both figures are, the better. It is worth restating that GI and GL are measures that relate to carbs. GI is not relevant to protein and fats, which is why none of the foods listed have a significant protein or fat content.

Let's take a quick look at breakfast:

FOOD	GI	GL	PORTION SIZE (OUNCES)
Oatmeal	50	10	1¾
Granola	43	7	1
Corn muffin	102	30	2
Bran muffin	60	15	2
Pancakes (buckwheat)	102	22	2⅝ (mix)
Bagel	72	25	2½
Cornflakes	80	20	1

Source: people.bu.edu/sobieraj/papers/GlycemicIndices.

You can see why, if you are having a carb breakfast, oatmeal and granola are better options than cornflakes or a bagel.

And what are you going to put on your granola?

FOOD	GI	GL	PORTION SIZE (OUNCES)
Milk, skim	27	3	8
Soy milk	44	8	8

The relatively high GI and GL of soy milk is just one reason to stick with dairy. And since we're handing out surprises, here's another one:

FOOD	GI	GL	PORTION SIZE (OUNCES)
Ice cream	37	4	1¾

You would bet your house on ice cream being high GI/GL, but not so. If you factor it into your calorie count, low-calorie ice cream with strawberries is a great treat to round off a meal. For more on the GI and GL of various foods and how best to plan your fast-day foods, see page 100.

What About Protein?

We certainly don't recommend eating protein to the exclusion of all else on a fast day, but you do require an adequate quantity for muscle health, cell maintenance, endocrinal regulation, immunity, and energy. Protein is satiating, too, so it's well worth including it in your calorie quota. The best advice is to stick to recommended USDA guidelines, which allow for a (quite generous) 50 grams (about 1¾ ounces) per day.

Go for "good protein." Steamed white fish, for example, is low in saturated fats and rich in minerals. Choose skinless chicken over red meat; try low-fat dairy products over endless lattes; include shrimp, tuna, and tofu or other plant-based proteins. Nuts, seeds, and legumes (beans, peas, and lentils) are full of fiber and act as bulking agents on a hungry day. Nuts, though high in calories (depending, of course, on how much you eat), are generally low GI and brilliantly satiating. They are fatty, too, so you might imagine they are "bad for you," yet the evidence is that nut consumers have lower rates of heart disease and diabetes than nut abstainers.[4]

Eggs, meanwhile, are low in saturated fat and full of nutritional value; they won't adversely affect your cholesterol levels, and they score a mere 90 calories each, so an egg-based breakfast on a fast day makes perfect sense. Two eggs plus a 1¾-ounce serving of smoked salmon clock in at a sensible 250 calories. Research recently found that individuals who consume egg protein for breakfast are more likely to feel full during the day than those whose breakfasts contain wheat protein.[5] Poaching or boiling an egg avoids the addition of careless calories. So give up the toast and replace it with steamed asparagus spears.

For more suggestions about foods to keep you full and fit on a fast day, and the benefits certain choices will bring, turn to page 100.

How to Fit Fasting into Your Life

When to Start?

If you do not have an underlying medical condition, and if you are not an individual for whom fasting is not advised (see page 115), then there really is no time like the present. Ask yourself: if not now, when? You may prefer to await a doctor's advice. You may choose to prepare yourself—to talk yourself down from a lifelong habit of overeating, to clear out the fridge, to eat the last cookie in the jar. Or you may want to get on with it and start to see visible progress within a couple of weeks. Do, however, begin on a day when you feel strong, purposeful, calm, and committed. Do tell friends and family that you're starting the FastDiet; once you make a public commitment, you are much more likely to stick with it. Avoid holidays, vacations, and days when you've got to attend a fancy business lunch complete with bread basket, cheese course, and four types of dessert. Recognize, too, that a busy day will help your fast time fly, while a lazy one generally goes as slow as molasses.

Once you've deliberated and designated a day to debut, get your mind in gear. Record your details—weight, BMI, target weight—in a diary before you start, and be ready to note your progress, knowing that dieters who keep an honest account of what they eat and drink are more likely to lose the pounds and keep them off. Then . . . take a deep breath and relax. Better yet, shrug. It's no big deal: you have nothing to lose but weight.

How Tough Will It Be?

If it has been a while since you have experienced hunger, even the slightest hint, you'll probably find that eating no more than 500 or 600 calories in a day is a mild challenge, at least initially. Intermittent fasters do report that the process becomes significantly easier with time, particularly as they witness results in the mirror and on the scale. Your first fast day should speed by, buoyed along by the novelty of the process; a fast day on a wet Wednesday in week three may feel more of a slog. Your mission is to complete it, knowing that although you are saying no to chocolate today, you will be eating what you want tomorrow. That is the joy of the FastDiet and what makes it so different from other weight-loss plans.

Although you are saying no to chocolate today, you will be eating what you want tomorrow. That is the joy of the FastDiet and what makes it so different from other weight-loss plans.

How to Win the Hunger Games

There is no reason to be alarmed by benign, occasional, short-term hunger. Given base-level good health, you will not perish. You won't collapse in a heap and need to be rescued by the cat. Your body is designed to go without food for longish periods, even if it has lost the skill through years of grazing, picking, and snacking. Research has found that modern humans tend to mistake a whole range of emotions for hunger.[6] We eat when we're bored, when we're thirsty, when we're around food (when aren't we?), when we're with company, or simply when the clock happens to tell us it's time for food. Most of us eat, too, just because it feels good. This is known as hedonic hunger, and while you should try to resist it on a fast day, you can bask in the knowledge that, if you please, you can give in to temptation the following day.

There's no need to panic about any of this. Simply note that the human brain is adept at persuading us that we're hungry in almost all situations: when faced with feelings of deprivation or withdrawal or disappointment; when angry, sad, happy, neutral; when subjected to advertising, social imperatives, sensory stimulation, reward, habit, the smell of freshly brewed coffee or bread baking or bacon cooking in a café up the road. Recognize now that these are often learned reactions to external cues, most of them designed to part you from your cash. If you are still processing your last meal, it's highly unlikely that what you are experiencing is true hunger ("total transit time," should you be interested in such things, can take up to two days, depending on your gender, your metabolism, and what you've eaten).

While hunger pangs can be aggressive and disagreeable, like a box of sharp knives, in practice they are more fluid and controllable than you might think. You're unlikely to be troubled at all by hunger until well into a fast day. What's more, a pang will pass. Fasters report that the feeling of perceived hunger comes in waves, not in an ever-growing wall of gnawing belly noise. It's a symphony of differentiated movements, not a steady, fearful crescendo. Treat a tummy rumble as a good sign, a healthy messenger.

Remember, too, that hunger does not build over a twenty-four-hour period, so don't feel trapped in the feeling at any given moment. Wait a while. You have absolute power to conquer feelings of hunger, simply by steering your mind, riding the wave, choosing to do something else—take a walk, phone a friend, drink tea, go for a run, take a shower, sing in the shower, phone a friend from the shower and sing . . . After a few weeks' practicing intermittent fasting, people generally report that their sense of hunger is diminished.

As we've seen, one of the key studies to investigate how obese subjects react to intermittent fasting was done with volunteers doing the more demanding alternate-day modified fasting method (ADMF) at the University of Illinois at Chicago. This study found that "during the first week of alternate-day modified fasting, hunger scores were elevated. However, after two weeks of ADMF, hunger scores decreased and remained low throughout the rest of the trial," demonstrating that "subjects become habituated to the ADMF diet (i.e., feel very little hunger on the fast day) after approximately two weeks." Furthermore, "satisfaction with the ADMF diet was low during the first four weeks of the intervention, but gradually increased during the last four weeks of the study." In short, the researchers concluded that "since hunger virtually diminishes, and since satisfaction with diet considerably increases within a short amount of time, it is likely that obese participants would be able to follow the diet for longer periods of time."[7] Remember, this research was done with people fasting every other day, something which we both tried and found challenging. By contrast partial fasting two days a week—the FastDiet plan—is a walk in the park.

So take heart. On a fast day, refrain, restrain, divert, and distract. Before you know it, you'll have retrained your brain and hunger's off the menu.

Tomorrow Is Another Day: Willpower, Patience, and Delayed Gratification

Perhaps the most reassuring and game-changing part of the FastDiet is that it doesn't last forever. Unlike deprivation diets that have failed you before, on this plan tomorrow will always be different. Easier. There may be pancakes for breakfast, or lunch with friends, wine with supper, apple pie with ice cream. This on/off switch is critical. It means that on a fast day, though you're eating a quarter of your usual calorie intake, tomorrow you can eat as you please. There's boundless psychological comfort in the fact that your fasting will only ever be a short stay, a brief break from food.

When you're not fasting, ignore fasting—it doesn't own you, it doesn't define you. You're not even doing it most of the time. Unlike full-time fad diets, you'll still get pleasure from food, you'll still have treats, you'll engage in the regular, routine, food-related events of your normal life. There are no special shakes, bars, rules, points, affectations, or idiosyncrasies. No saying "no" all the time. For this reason, you won't feel serially deprived, which—as anyone who has embarked on the grinding chore of long-term everyday dieting knows—is precisely why conventional diet plans fail.

> Unlike full-time fad diets, you'll still get pleasure from food, you'll still have treats, you'll engage in the regular, routine, food-related events of your normal life.

The key, then, is to recognize, through patience and the exercise of will, that you can make it through to breakfast tomorrow. Bear in mind that fasting subjects regularly report that the food with which they "break their fast" tastes glorious. Flavors sing. Mouthfuls dance. If you've ever felt a lazy disregard for the food you consume without thinking, then things are about to change. There's nothing like a bit of delayed gratification to make things taste good.

Compliance and Sustainability: How to Discover a Sensible Eating Pattern That Works for You

Most diets don't work. You know that already. Indeed, when a team of psychologists at UCLA conducted an analysis of thirty-one long-term diet trials back in 2007, they concluded that "several studies indicate that dieting is a consistent predictor of future weight gain . . . We asked what evidence is there that dieting works in the long term, and found that the evidence shows the opposite." Their analysis found that while dieters do lose pounds in the early months, the vast majority return to their original weight within five years, while "at least a third end up heavier than when they embarked on the project."[8] The standard approach clearly hasn't worked, doesn't work, and won't work.

In order to be effective, then, any method must be rational, sustainable, flexible, and feasible over the long haul. Adherence, not weight loss per se, is the key, so your goals must be realistic and the program practical. It must fit into your life as it is, not the life of your dreams. It needs to go on vacation with you, it needs to visit friends, get you through a boring day at the office, and cope with Christmas. To work at all, any weight-loss strategy has to be tolerable, organic, and innate, not some spurious add-on that makes you feel awkward and self-conscious, the dietary equivalent of uncomfortable shoes.

While the long-term experience of intermittent fasters is still under investigation, people who have tried it comment on how easily it fits into everyday life. They still get variety from food (anyone who's ever tried to lose weight on only grapefruit or cabbage soup will know how vital this is). They still get rewards from food. They still get a life. There is no drama, no desperate dieting, no self-flagellation. No sweat.

Flexibility: Your Key to Success

Your body is not my body. Mine is not yours. So it's worth carving out your plan according to your needs, the shape of your day, your family, your commitments, your preferences. None of us live cookie-cutter lives, and no single diet plan fits all. Everyone has quirks and qualifiers. That's why there are no absolute commandments here, just suggestions. You may choose to fast in a particular way, on a particular day. You may like to eat once, or twice, first thing or last. You may like beets or fennel or blueberries. Some individuals prefer to be told exactly what to eat and when; others like a more informal approach. That's fine. It's enough to simply stick to the basic method—500 or 600 calories a day, with as long a window without food as possible, twice a week—and you'll gain the plan's multiple benefits. In time, there's little need for assiduous calorie counting; you'll know what a fast day means and how it best suits you.

The Maintenance Model

Once you've reached your target weight or just a shade below (allowing room for flexibility and a generous slice of birthday cake), you may consider adopting the Maintenance Model. This is an adjustment to fasting in which you fast on only one day each week in order to remain in a holding pattern at your desired weight but still reap the antiaging benefits of occasional fasting. Naturally, one day a week—if that's what you choose—may offer fewer health benefits in the long run than two; but it does fit neatly into your life, particularly if you are not intent on achieving any further weight loss. Equally, if the beach beckons or there's a wedding on the calendar or you've woken up on the day after Christmas haunted by that fourth roast potato, step it back up. You're in charge.

What To Expect

The first thing you can expect from adopting the FastDiet, of course, is to lose weight—some weeks more, some weeks less; some weeks finding yourself stuck at a disappointing plateau, other weeks making swifter progress. As a basic guide, you might anticipate a loss of around a pound with each fast day. This will not, of course, be all fat. Some will be water, and some the digested food in your system. You should, however, lose around ten pounds of fat over a ten-week period, which beats a typical low-calorie diet. Crucially, you can expect to maintain your weight loss over time.

More important than what you'll lose, though, is what you're set to gain.

How Your Anatomy Will Change

Over a period of weeks, you can expect your BMI, body fat percentage, and waist measurement to drop and your lean muscle mass to increase. Your cholesterol count, blood glucose, and IGF-1 levels will improve. This is the path to greater health and extended life. You are already dodging your unwritten future. Right now, though, the palpable changes will start to show up in the mirror as your body becomes leaner and lighter.

> Over a period of weeks, you can expect your BMI, body fat percentage, and waist measurement to drop and your lean muscle mass to increase. Your cholesterol count, blood glucose, and IGF-1 levels will improve.

As the weeks progress, you'll find that intermittent fasting has potent secondary effects, too. Alongside the obvious weight loss and health benefits stored up for the future, there are more subtle consequences, perks, and bonuses that can come into play.

How Your Appetite Will Change

Expect your food preferences to adapt; pretty soon, you'll start to choose healthy foods by default, not by design. You will begin to understand hunger, to negotiate and manage it, knowing how it feels to be properly hungry. You'll also recognize the sensation of being pleasantly full, not groaning like an immovable sofa. Satiated, not stuffed. The upshot? No more "food hangovers," improved digestion, more bounce.

After six months of intermittent fasting, interesting things should happen to your eating habits. You may find that you eat half the meat you once did—not as a conscious move, but a natural one born of what you desire rather than what you decide or believe. You're likely to consume more vegetables. Many intermittent fasters instinctively retreat from bread (and, by association, butter), while stodgy "comfort" foods seem less appealing and refined sugars aren't nearly as tempting as they once were. The bag of candy in the glove compartment of the car? Take it or leave it.

Of course, you don't need to dwell actively on any of this. If you are like me, then one day soon, you'll arrive at a place where you say no to the cheesecake because you don't want it, not because you are denying yourself a treat. This is the baseline power of intermittent fasting: it encourages you to recheck your diet. And that's your long-haul ticket to health.

How Your Attitude Will Change

So yes, you'll start to lose bad habits around food. But if you continue to fast—and feast—with awareness, all kinds of other changes should occur, some of them unlikely and unexpected. You may, for instance, discover that you've been suffering from "portion distortion" for years, thinking that the food piled on your plate is the quantity you really need and want. With time, you'll probably discover that you've been overdoing it. Muffins will start to look vast as they sit, fat and moist, under glass domes in the coffee shops. A large bag of chips becomes a monstrous prospect. You may go from venti to grande to only wanting half a cup, no sugar, no cream.

Soon you'll come to recognize the truth about how you've been eating and the wordless fibs you've told yourself for years. This is as much a part of the recalibrating process as anything else; you've changed your mind. Occasional fasting will train you in the art of "restrained eating"; at the end of the day, this is the goal. It's all part of the long game of behavioral change that means that the FastDiet will ultimately become neither a fast nor a diet, but a way of life. After a while, you'll have cultivated a new approach to eating—thoughtful, rational, responsible—without even knowing you're doing it.

Intermittent fasters also report a boost to their energy, together with an amplified sense of emotional well-being. Some talk of a "glow"—the result, perhaps, of winning the battle for self-control, or from the smaller clothes and the compliments, or from something going on at a metabolic level that governs our moods. We may not yet know precisely why, but whatever it is, it feels good. Far better than cake. As one online devotee says, "Overall, fasting just seems right. It's like a reset button for your entire body."[9]

More subtly still, many fasters acknowledge a sense of relief as their fast days no longer revolve around food. Embrace it. There's a certain liberty here, if you allow it to materialize. You may find, as we have, that you start to look forward to your fasts: a time to regroup and give feeding a rest.

And now, on to the FastDiet in reality: tales, tips, and troubleshooting.

How Men Fast:
Michael's Experience

A lot of men have contacted me over the last few months to let me know how much weight they have lost and also how surprised and delighted they are that intermittent fasting turns out to be so easy. They like its simplicity, the fact that you don't have to give things up or try to remember complicated recipes. I also think they rather like the challenge.

The British actor and comedian Dom Joly recently wrote that he'd lost thirty-five pounds after watching my *Horizon* program and felt it was an approach he could imagine sticking to for the rest of his life.[10] The attraction for him is that he knows he will be able to eat what he wants the following day. He even added that he now rather enjoys the fasting days, something I have heard from a number of men. One of the things that men seem to like particularly about fasting is that they can fit it into their lives with minimal hassle. It doesn't stop them working, traveling, socializing, or exercising. In fact, some find it fuels performance (see page 113 for more on fasting and exercise).

In one Belgian study, men asked to eat a high-fat diet and exercise before breakfast on an empty stomach put on far less weight than a similar group of men on an identical diet who exercised after breakfast.[11] This study adds support to the claim that eating in a fasted state makes the body burn a greater percentage of fat for fuel. At least it does if you are a man.

For me, a fast day now follows a familiar routine. I start with a protein-rich breakfast, normally scrambled eggs or a dish of cottage cheese. I drink several cups of black coffee and tea during the day, work happily through lunch, and rarely feel any hunger pangs until well into the late afternoon. When they happen, I simply ignore them or go for a brief stroll until they pass.

In the evening I have a bit of meat or fish and piles of steamed vegetables. Having abstained since breakfast, I find them particularly delicious. I never have problems getting to sleep and most days wake up the next morning feeling no more peckish than normal.

How Women Fast:
Mimi's Experience

While most men I know respond well to numbers and targets (with associated gadgets, if at all possible), I've found that women tend to take a more holistic approach to fasting. As with much in life, we like to examine how it feels, knowing that our bodies are unique and will respond to any given stimulation in their own sweet way. We respond to shared stories and the support of friends. And, sometimes, we need a snack.

Personally, for instance, I like to consume my fast-day calories in two lots—one early, one late—bookending the day with my allowance and aiming for a longish gap in between to maximize the prospect of health gains and weight loss. But I do need a little something to keep me going in between. A fast-day breakfast is usually a low-sugar muesli, perhaps including some fresh strawberries and almonds, with 1% or 2% milk; there'll be an apple for lunch—hardly a feast, I know, but just enough to make a difference to the day. Then, supper: a substantial, interesting salad with heaps of leaves and some lean protein—perhaps smoked salmon or tuna or hummus—once the kids are in bed. Throughout the day, I drink mineral water with a squeeze of lime, tons of herbal tea, and plenty of black coffee. They just help the day tick by.

In the four months since I started the FastDiet, I have lost 13.2 pounds, and my BMI has gone from 21.4 to 19.4.

If you're struggling with bigger numbers than these, take strength from the fact that heavier subjects respond brilliantly to intermittent fasting, and the positive effects should be apparent in a relatively short time. These days, one fast a week (on Mondays) seems to suffice and keep me at a stable, happy weight.

Many women I encounter are well versed in dieting techniques (years of practice), and I've found a couple of tips that come in handy on a fast day. I recommend, for instance, eating in small mouthfuls, chewing slowly, and concentrating when eating. Why read a magazine, why tweet as you eat? If you're getting only 500 calories, it makes sense to notice them as they go in.

Like many intermittent fasters, I have found that hunger is simply not an issue. For whatever reason—and one wonders whether it suits the food industry—we have developed a fear of hunger, fretting about low blood sugar and whatnot. On the whole, for me, a day with little food feels emancipated rather than restrictive. That said, there are ups and downs: some days skip by like a pebble on water; other days, I feel like I'm sinking, not swimming, perhaps because emotions or hormones or simply the tricky business of life have kicked in. See how you feel, and always give in gracefully if that particular day is not your day to fast.

A Dozen Ways to Make the FastDiet Work for You

1. Know your weight and your BMI from the get-go. As we mentioned earlier, one of the best things you can do is calculate your body mass index—your weight (in pounds) divided by your height (in inches) squared, multiplied by a conversion factor of 703; it may sound like palaver, and an abstract one at that, but it's the best tool we have to plot a path to healthy weight loss. (Or you can just let a BMI website do the calculation.) Do note that a BMI score takes no account of body type, age, or ethnicity, and so should be greeted with informed caution. Still, if you need a number, this is the one to watch.

Weigh yourself regularly but not obsessively. Once a week should suffice. The mornings after fast days are best if you like to see falling figures. Researchers at the University of Illinois have noted that "weight measurements are drastically different from feed to fast day. This discrepancy in body weight is most likely due to the additional weight of food present in the gastrointestinal tract, and not changes in fat mass from day to day. As a potential solution, future trials should average body weight measurements taken from consecutive feed and fast days to attain a more accurate assessment of weight."[12] You might like to do the same, but don't make weighing—yourself or your food—a chore. If you are someone who enjoys structure and clarity, you may want to monitor your progress. Have a target in mind. Where do you want to be, and when? Be realistic: precipitous weight loss is not advised, so allow yourself time. Make a plan. Write it down.

Plenty of people recommend keeping a diet diary. Alongside the numbers, add your experiences; try to note down "Three Good Things" that happen on that day. It's a feel-good message that you can refer to as time goes by.

2. **Find a fast friend.** You need very few accoutrements to make this a success, but a supportive friend may well be one of them. Once you're on the FastDiet, tell people about it; you may find that they join in, and you'll develop a network of common experience. Since the plan appeals to men and women equally, couples report that they find it more manageable to do it together. That way you get mutual support, camaraderie, joint commitment, and shared anecdotes; besides, mealtimes are made infinitely easier if you're eating with someone who understands the rudiments of the plot. There are plenty of threads on online chat rooms and forums, which are great sources

of support and information. It's remarkable how reassuring it is to know that you're not alone.

3. **Prep your fast-day food in advance** so that you don't go foraging and come across a leftover sausage lurking irresistibly in the fridge. Keep it simple, aiming for fast-day flavor without effort. Shop and cook on nonfast days instead, so as not to taunt yourself with undue temptation (for simple, sustaining fast-day recipe ideas, see chapter 3). Before you embark on the FastDiet, clear the house of junk food. It will only croon and coo at you from the cupboard, making your fast day harder than it needs to be.

4. **Check calorie labels for portion size**. When the cereal box says "a 30g serving," weigh it out. Go on. Be amazed. Then be honest. Since your calorie count on a fast day is necessarily fixed and limited, it's important not to be blinkered about how much is actually going in. You'll find a calorie counter for suggested fast-day foods starting on page 171. Or download a calorie counter app such as www.myfitnesspal.com. For more detailed information, try www.nutritiondata.self.com, which includes specific search criteria to allow you to fit your food choices not only to your calorie allocation but also to your nutritional needs. Way more

important: don't count calories on a nonfast day. You've got better things to do.

5. **Wait before you eat**. Try to resist for at least ten minutes, fifteen if you can, to see if the hunger subsides (as it naturally tends to do). If you absolutely must snack, choose something that will not elevate your insulin levels. Try some carrot sticks, a handful of plain air-popped popcorn, an apple slice, or some strawberries. But don't pick and peck like a hen through the day; the calories will soon stack up and your fast will be dashed. On fast days, eat with awareness, allowing yourself to fully absorb the fact that you're eating (not as daft as it sounds, particularly if you have ever sat in a traffic jam popping M&M's). Similarly, on off-duty days, stay gently alert. Eat until you're satisfied, not until you're full (this will come naturally after a few weeks' practice). Work out what the concept of "fullness" means for you—we are all different, and it changes over time.

6. **Stay busy.** "We humans are always looking for things to do between meals," said singer-songwriter Leonard Cohen. Yes, and look where it's got us. So fill your day, not your face. As fasting advocate Brad Pilon has noted, "No one's hungry in the first few seconds of a skydive." Engage in things other

than food—not necessarily skydiving, but anything that appeals to you. Distraction is your best defense against the dark arts of the food industry, which has stationed doughnuts on every street corner and nachos at every turn. And remember, if you must have that doughnut, it will still be there tomorrow.

7. **Try the two-to-two,** fasting not from bedtime to bedtime, but from 2:00 p.m. until 2:00 p.m. After lunch on day one, eat sparingly until a late lunch the following day. That way, you lose weight as you sleep and no single day feels uncomfortably deprived of food. It's a clever trick, but it does require a modicum more concentration than the whole-day option. Or perhaps fast from supper to supper, which again means that no day is "all fast and no fun." The point is that this plan is "adjust to fit." Just like your waistband in three weeks' time.

8. **Don't be afraid to think about food you like.** A psychological mechanism called habituation—in which the more people have of something, the less value they attach to it—means that doing the opposite and trying to suppress thoughts of food is a flawed strategy.[13] The critical thought process here is to treat food as a friend, not a foe. Food is

not magical, supernatural, or dangerous. Don't demonize it; normalize it. It's only food.

9. **Stay hydrated.** Find no-calorie drinks you like, and then drink them in quantity. Some swear by herbal tea, others prefer mineral water with bubbles to dance on the tongue, though tap water will do just as well. Plenty of our hydration comes through the food we eat, so fasters may need to compensate with additional drinks beyond their routine intake (check your urine; it should be plentiful and pale). While there's no scientific rationale for drinking the recommended eight glasses of water a day, there is good reason to keep the liquids coming in. A dry mouth is the last sign of dehydration, not the first, so act before your body complains, recognizing too that a glass of water is a quick way to hush an empty belly, at least temporarily. It will also stop you from mistaking thirst for hunger.

10. **Don't count on weight loss on any given day.** If you have a week when the scale doesn't seem to shift, dwell instead upon the health benefits you will certainly be accruing even if you haven't seen your numbers drop. Remember why you're doing this: not just the smaller jeans, but the long-term advantages: the widely accepted disease-busting, brain-boosting, life-lengthening benefits of intermittent fasting. Think of it as a pension plan for your body.

11. **Be sensible, exercise caution, and if it feels wrong, stop**. It's vital that this strategy should be practiced in a way that's flexible and forgiving. It's okay to break the rules if you need to. It's not a race to the finish, so be kind and make it fun. Who wants to live longer if it's in abject misery? You don't want to grunt and sweat under a weary life. You want to go dancing. Right?

12. **Congratulate yourself**. Every completed fast day means potential weight loss and quantifiable health gain. You're already winning.

Q & A

Which days should I choose to fast?

It really doesn't matter. It's your life, and you'll know which days will suit you best. Monday is an obvious choice for many, perhaps because it is more manageable, psychologically and practically, to gear yourself up at the beginning of a new week, particularly if it follows a sociable weekend. For that reason, fasters might choose to avoid Saturdays and Sundays, when family lunches and brunches, dinner dates and parties make calorie-cutting a chore. Thursday would then make a sensible second fasting day. But be flexible; don't force yourself to fast when it feels wrong. If you're particularly stressed, off-kilter, tired, or peevish on a day that you have designated a fast, try again another day. Adapt. This is not about one-size-fits-all rules; it's about finding a realistic pattern that works for you. Do, however, aim for a pattern. That way, over time your fasts will become familiar, a low-key habit you accept and embrace. You may adapt your fasts as your life—and your body— change shape. But don't drop too many fast days; there is a danger that you'll slide back into old habits. Be kind. But be tough.

Does it have to be for twenty-four hours?

Fasting for a twenty-four-hour period is practical, coherent, and unambiguous, all of which will promise a greater chance of success. It is, however, only the most convenient way of organizing a fast. There's nothing magical about twenty-four hours. To save on bother, stick to it, and remind yourself that you'll be asleep for nearly a third of it.

Should I fast on consecutive days?

Most of the human studies done to date have involved volunteers fasting on consecutive days; there may be some value in doing back-to-back fasts, but as far as we are aware, there are no human studies comparing this approach with split fast days. We do, however, know what works in practice for many fasters. Michael tried the consecutive system and found it too challenging to be sustainable over time, so he switched to the split version—fasting on Mondays and Thursdays. The weight loss, improvements in glucose, cholesterol, and IGF-1 that he saw are all the result of this nonconsecutive two-day pattern.

There's a psychological imperative here, too: fast for more than a day at a time, and you may start to feel resentful, bored, and beleaguered—precisely the feelings that wreck the best-made diet intentions. A critical part of this plan is that you never feel challenged for long enough to consider quitting. By the time you've had enough, breakfast is on the table and another fast has passed.

How much weight will I lose?

This will depend largely on your own metabolism, your individual body type, your starting weight, your level of activity, and how effectively and honestly you fast. In the first week, you may experience water loss that can account for a significant dip on the scale; with time, your weekly calorie deficit will mean, thanks to the simple law of thermogenics (weight loss occurs when energy in is less than energy out), that you will be losing fat. Be judicious: abrupt weight loss is not advised and shouldn't be your aim. You may, however, anticipate losing around seven pounds in eight weeks.

I know I should stick to low-GI or low-GL foods on a fast day. So which foods are best?

As we've seen, foods with a low glycemic index or glycemic load will help keep your blood sugars stable, increasing your chances of a successful day with few calories. Vegetables and legumes are, needless to say, amazing, and you should rely on them on a fast day. Packed with nutrients, their bulk fills you up, they have relatively few calories, and they keep your blood sugar low. Carrots are a great snack, particularly with hummus dip, which scores an astonishing GI of 6 and 0 on the GL score. Fruit is handy too, though some fruits are more fast-friendly than others.

Check the GI count of your chosen fast-day foods online. The American Diabetes Association has an excellent guide on its website under "Glycemic Index and Diabetes." Staple starchy foods, for instance, are worth scrutinizing with an eagle eye:

FOOD	GI	GL	PORTION SIZE (OUNCES)
Brown rice	48	20	5¼
White rice	76	36	5¼
Pasta (durum wheat)	40	20	5¼
Couscous	65	23	5¼
Potatoes, boiled	58	16	5¼
Potatoes, mashed	85	17	5¼
Potatoes, fried	75	22	5¼
Potatoes, baked	85	26	5¼

The biggest surprise among the staples is how big an effect baked or mashed potatoes have on blood sugars. On fast days, avoid these starchy basics and substitute plenty of greens. Fill your plate. Watch out for fruit, too. Some are your fast friends, but others will spike your blood sugar and are best left for the days when you are eating freely.

FOOD	GI	GL	PORTION SIZE (OUNCES)
Strawberries	38	1	4¼
Apples	35	5	4¼
Oranges	42	5	4¼
Grapes	45	9	4¼
Pineapple	84	7	4¼
Banana	50	12	4¼
Raisins	64	30	2
Dates	100	42	2

Eating the whole fruit will keep you feeling full for longer. Strawberries, without sugar, are extraordinarily low GI/GL and also low in calories; no wonder many fasters eat a bowl for breakfast. The striking thing to note is the high sugar impact of raisins and dates. Avoid them on fast days. For calorie counts, turn to the Calorie Counter on page 171.

Eating the whole fruit will keep you feeling full for longer.

I've read about "super foods" and "intelligent eating." Should I include super foods during a fast day?

The term "super food" is more of a marketing ploy than a scientific construct, and clinical nutritionists are loath to use the description. Still, there is evidence to suggest that some foods are rich in nutrients or phytochemicals that can have a beneficial role in the body. If you like them, eat them— on a fast day or, indeed, on any day you please. They can't hurt, they taste good, and they're generally fresh and low in calories—making them ideal fast-day companions.

Fruit: As the labs of the world continue in their quest for new antiobesity marvels, the latest to emerge is the humble tangerine. Citrus fruits in general, and tangerines in particular, contain high concentrations of nobiletin, a compound that "protects from obesity and atherosclerosis"—in lab mice at least.[14] If you like tangerines, eat them, perhaps spending time meditatively peeling away the pith. The same group of researchers previously found that grapefruit, rich in a compound called naringenin, encourages the liver to burn fat rather than store it.[15] Grapefruit also contains compounds such as liminoids and lycopene (thought to have anticancer properties),[16] and clocks in at only 39 calories per half, making it a good fast-day food. (You should, however, be aware that grapefruit interacts with a number of common medicines, so if you are taking medication such as statins, consult your doctor.) Alternatively, you could always throw in a watermelon slice (30 calories per 100 grams, about 3½ ounces) or an apple (around 50 calories per 100 grams) for flavor, crunch, and pectin, a soluble fiber that can't be absorbed by the body but is useful in fat digestion.[17] Apples are the ultimate convenience food, though they are quite high in calories; eat the whole thing, skin, seeds, and core—you'll probably want to if it's one of your fast-day treats. Tomatoes also contain lycopene, which may help guard against cancer[18] and stroke.[19] A handful of cherry tomatoes or strawberries (low GI, low GL) could be your best bet to get you through a tummy rumble unscathed. Check for calorie traps before you eat (see the Calorie Counter on page 171).

Berries: Blueberries are high in antioxidant polyphenols and phytonutrients. New research has found that these bold little berries may also be able to break down fat cells in the body and prevent new ones from forming.[20] Pretty impressive, eh? Even if you don't buy the science, blueberries remain a handy source of vitamin C. Once you're berry savvy, you may want to cruise your local health food store for other super foods: goji, açai, aloe, hemp seeds, chia seeds, and spirulina (a nutrient-rich blue-green algae). All curious, all good.

Vegetables: Again, aim for a wide variety of vegetation—different colors, textures, tastes, shapes. Steamed broccoli contains a whole world of nutrients (including vitamin K). Green beans love a little lemon and garlic. Fennel is great if shaved (invest in a mandoline), perhaps teamed with orange segments and a squeeze of the juice. Edamame is a good source of low-fat protein and omega-3 fatty acids.

Starchy veggies, of course, tend to have a higher GL and calorific value, though they are satiating. Proceed with caution and don't add butter.

Leaves: It goes without saying that green leafy veggies are your fast-day friends. Spinach, kale, chard, mustard greens, salad leaves . . . a veritable vitamin fest, and agreeably low in calories. Pep things up with chili flakes, ginger, cumin, pepper, lemon juice, garlic. Garlic, by the way, contains allicin, the active ingredient that lends it pungency and is also thought to protect cells and reduce fatty deposits,[21] so be liberal and carry (sugarless) mints.

Herbs and spices: Lo-cal, high-impact, no brainer. Pickles may work for you too—cornichons, jalapeños, onions (watch the GI values)—or mustard; anything, really, that brings a bolt of fire or flavor to your plate.

Nuts: We've established that nuts are a fast-day favorite: filling and low GI. Almonds, though calorific, are high in protein and fiber, which makes them brilliantly satiating; pistachios, too (better yet, they take ages to crack and eat). Cashews and coconut flakes will help animate a salad. But count wisely; nut calories soon add up.

Seeds: Sunflower seeds contain good fats, together with iron, zinc, potassium, vitamins E and B_1, magnesium, and selenium—all that goodness in a tiny little packet.

Soup: Scientists at Penn State University have found that soup is a great appetite suppressant.[22] Go for a light broth or a miso soup; choose carrot and coriander over a creamy chowder.

Cereals: Oats are a standby low-GL staple, but mix it up;

you could experiment with bulgur, couscous, or quinoa—they're high in protein and fiber, easy to cook, and a good source of iron.

Dairy: Milk products, though full of protein and calcium, can also be high in fat. Opt for low-fat alternatives—and save the cheese board for tomorrow. Fat-free yogurt will bring protein, potassium, and—if you want them—probiotics along to the party, and like nuts, will help you feel fuller longer.

Whatever you eat on a fast day (or any day), the most important thing is to relish it. Go slow. Have a look at the menu plans starting on page 127 for more ideas.

> Whatever you eat on a fast day (or any day), the most important thing is to relish it. Go slow.

I know I need plenty of veggies, but should I eat them raw or cooked?

There is some debate as to whether vegetables are best eaten raw or cooked; cooking may, as raw foodists contend, destroy vitamins, minerals, and enzymes, but it also softens cellulose fibers, making nutrients more available for take-up in the body. Lycopene, a potent antioxidant found in tomatoes, is boosted in cooking.[23] A small blob of ketchup is no bad thing. Meanwhile, boiled or steamed carrots, spinach, mushrooms, asparagus, cabbage, peppers, and many other vegetables supply more antioxidants, such as carotenoids and ferulic acid, to the body than they do when raw.[24] The downside of cooking vegetables is that it can destroy their vitamin C. The raw versus cooked argument is a complicated one. Our best advice? Eat plenty of vegetables, just the way you like them.

Can I really eat what I like on the off-duty days?

Yes. Counterintuitive as it may seem, no foods are off-limits, none forbidden. On the five days a week when we're not restricting calories, we both eat freely—fish and chips, roast potatoes, cookies, cake. The Illinois study certainly found that volunteers encouraged to eat lasagna, pizza, and fries during "off days" still lost weight.

Even so, don't *try* to gorge in a bid to make up for lost time, like a contestant in a blueberry pie–eating contest. You could compensate for fasting by grossly overeating the next day, but it's very hard to do and you probably won't want to; a calorie slash of 75 percent on a fast day generally gives rise to little more than a 15 percent increase on the following feed day.

This absence of hyperphagia (excessive appetite) on a nonfast day surprised the research team: "We hypothesized that the participants would increase their energy intake on the feed day by approximately 125% of their baseline needs. However, no such hyperphagic response was observed . . . on average, subjects were only consuming 95 (± 6)% of their calculated energy needs on the feed day. This change in meal pattern helped these subjects to achieve a marked degree of energy restriction (37% net daily), which was related to the pronounced weight loss attained (5.6 kg [12.32 pounds] in eight weeks). These preliminary data suggest that subjects are not likely to consume higher fat diets on the feed day when partaking in an ADMF regimen."[25]

Humans have, however, evolved to prefer calorie-rich foods—it once gave us an edge—and perhaps the greatest advantage of the FastDiet is that it includes pleasure foods on five days of the week. For most of the time, there is no limitation, no deprivation, no guilt. The psychological impact of *not* being in denial is huge; it frustrates what's known as the "disinhibition effect"—a paradox where designating certain foods off-limits makes us likely to eat more of them.[26]

Remember, then, that this is not a cycle of bingeing and starving: it is calibrated and moderate. Studies and experience show that intermittent fasting will regulate the appetite, not make it more extreme. You could pig out on your nonfast days, working your way steadily through all the ice cream flavors in the freezer (even if you did, you'd still get some of the metabolic benefits of fasting). But you won't do that. In all likelihood, you'll remain gently, intuitively attentive to your calorie intake, almost without noticing. Similarly, you may find yourself naturally favoring healthier foods once your palate is modified by your occasional fasts. So yes, eat freely, forbid nothing, but trust your body to say "when."

Is breakfast important?

Dieting lore has long suggested that breakfast is the most important meal of the day—miss it in the morning and it's like leaving the house without a coat. But that's not necessarily the case. Recent research shows that a bigger breakfast begets a bigger lunch (and a bigger dinner), which—no surprises here—means a higher overall calorie count for the day.[27] Some fasters find that they need sustenance to start the day; others may prefer to wait to "break their fast" until later. It's up to you, and whichever pattern you choose may change over time.

What can I drink?

Plenty—as long as it doesn't carry a substantial calorie content. In practice, as with most decisions on the FastDiet, the choice is entirely up to you. Drink plenty of water—it's calorie-free, *actually* free, more filling than you think, and will stop you from confusing thirst for hunger. In summer, add rounds of cucumber or a dash of lime. Freeze it and suck on cubes. If you want warmth, miso soup contains protein, feels like food, and clocks in at only about 40 calories per cup; vegetable bouillon pulls off the same trick. A mug of instant low-cal hot chocolate, made with water? Under 40 calories and a comforting thought. No-cal drinks are better still. Hot water with lemon is a standby favorite for fasters, but you might prefer to add mint leaves or a scattering of cloves, a slice of ginger, or some lemongrass. If you are fond of herbal teas, try some unfamiliar flavors to spice up the day (licorice and cinnamon, lemongrass and ginger, lavender, rose and chamomile . . .). Green tea may have health-giving antioxidant properties (the jury's out), but if you like it, drink it. Remember that tea and coffee should be black and sugarless. Fruit juices generally have a surprisingly high sugar content, are lower in fiber than a whole fruit, and can rack up the stealth calories without so much as a by-your-leave. Commercial smoothies can have a sugar content similar to Coke and are loaded with calories; and because they are acidic, they are corrosive to your teeth. If you need flavor, swap out juice and smoothies for very dilute nonalcoholic spritzers—perhaps club soda with a dash of cranberry juice cocktail and lots of ice.

What about alcohol?

Alcoholic drinks, though pleasant, merely provide empty calories. One glass of white wine contains about 120 calories, while a 12-ounce can of beer racks up 153. Unless you really can't say no, abstain absolutely on a fast day—it's a golden opportunity to slash your weekly consumption without feeling deprived. Think of it as going cold turkey for two achievable days each week.

And caffeine?

There's a growing body of evidence to suggest that far from being a guilty pleasure, drinking coffee may be good for you, helping to prevent mental decline, improve cardiac health, and reduce the risk of liver cancer and stroke.[28] So go ahead, drink coffee if that's what gets you going and keeps you going each day. It's a useful weapon in your arsenal against boredom, and a coffee break makes a happy punctuation to the day. There's no metabolic reason to avoid caffeine during a fast, but if you have trouble sleeping, limit your intake later in the day. You should, of course, drink it black. A sixteen-ounce caramel macchiato has 224 calories . . . just saying.

How about snacks?

The general idea of the FastDiet is to give your body an occasional holiday from eating. Let your mouth rest. Give your belly a break. If you must snack on a fast day, do it with awareness and frugality, always keeping an eye on the GI.

FOOD	GI	GL	PORTION SIZE (OUNCES)
Nuts	27	3	1¾
Popcorn	72	8	⅔
Rice cakes	80	19	⅞
Fruit bars	93	20	1
Mars bar	65	26	2

You knew that chocolate bars were hardly a health food, but did you know how sugary fruit bars and even some rice cakes can be? Bear in mind that processed foods tend to have hidden sugars and, though convenient, won't give you anything like the nutritional advantage of good old-fashioned plants and proteins. Try carrot or celery sticks with hummus, or a handful of nuts—always factoring them into your daily calorie count (don't cheat).

Habitual snacking, even on low-calorie, nutrient-rich foods, is not advised; part of the motive here is to retrain your appetite, so don't overstimulate it. If your mouth is desperate for attention, give it a drink.

What are the implications of cheating and having a few chips or a cookie?

To clarify: this is a book about fasting, the voluntary abstention from eating food. The reasons this is good for you go way beyond the fact that you are simply eating fewer calories. The benefits arise because our bodies are designed for intermittent fasts. As you've seen, the scientific term is hormesis; what does not kill you makes you stronger. So while starvation is bad, a little bit of short, sharp, shock food restriction is good.

Your aim, then, is to carve out a food-free breathing space for your body. Going to 510 calories (or 615 for a man) won't hurt—it won't obliterate the fast. Indeed, the idea of slashing calories to a quarter of your daily intake on a fast day is simply one that has been clinically proven to have systemic effects on the metabolism. While there's no particular magic to 500 or 600 calories, do try to stick resolutely to these numbers; you need clear parameters to make the strategy effective in the medium term.

Having an extra cookie on a fast day would be antithetical to your goals (not to mention the fact that it would probably spike your blood sugar and eat up most of your allowance in one buttery bite); when you're fasting, you need to think sensibly and coherently about your food choices, following the plan laid out here. Exercise willpower, reminding yourself that tomorrow is on its way.

Can I use meal replacement shakes to get me through the early days?

A number of people who have tried fasting say that commercially available meal replacement shakes helped them get through the first, and normally hardest, weeks of an intermittent fast. Shakes are simpler than calorie counting, and on your fast day you simply sip away when waves of hunger strike. We are not great fans, as we think real food is better, but if you find they help, then by all means use them. It's best to go for a brand that is low in sugar.

Should I take supplements during my fast?

The FastDiet is an intermittent method, not a deprivation regimen, so your nutritional intake from a wide variety of food sources should remain relatively steady over time, providing all the vitamins and minerals you require. If, as recommended, your fast-day foods center on protein and plants, they'll give you all the goodness you need without resorting to costly bottled multivitamins. Do, however, choose your fast-day foods with care, ensuring that over the course of a week you consume adequate B vitamins, omega-3s, calcium, and iron. Be sensible and eat well. While we are no fans of bottled vitamins and minerals, if a qualified health professional has suggested a particular supplement, you should continue to take it.

Should I exercise on a fast day?

Why not? In the interests of flexibility and normality, there's no reason to change your usual pattern of activity while fasting. Research demonstrates that even a more extreme three-day total fast has no negative effect on the ability to perform short-term, high-intensity workouts or long-duration, moderate-intensity exercise. Athletes seem to suffer no loss in performance during occasional fasting; a 2008 study of Tunisian soccer players during Ramadan found that fasting had no effect on performance ("Each player was assessed for speed, power, agility, endurance, and for passing and dribbling skills. No variables were negatively affected by fasting."[29]) In fact—and this is worth noting if you are aiming for optimal fitness—fasted training can result in better metabolic adaptations[30] (which means enhanced performance over time), improved muscle protein synthesis,[31] and a higher anabolic response to post-exercise feeding.[32]

Training on an empty stomach turns out to be beneficial on multiple levels, coaxing the body to burn a greater percentage of fat for fuel instead of relying on recently consumed carbs; if you're burning fat, don't forget, you're not storing it. As we've seen, one recent study found that working out before breakfast is beneficial for metabolic performance and weight loss.[33] That same study, reports *The New York Times*, indicates that prebreakfast exercise "blunts the deleterious effects of overindulging"—making fasted exercise a handy way of "combating Christmas."[34] According to the study's authors, "Our current data indicate that exercise training in the fasted state is more effective than exercise in the carbohydrate-fed state." Certainly food for thought.

Are there gender differences in response to intermittent fasting?

Clearly, men and women have metabolic and hormonal differences; for evolutionary reasons, we store and utilize fat in different ways. Women carry more fat, are better at storing it, and tend to be more efficient at burning fat in response to exercise.[35]

Though few studies have been done, there's some evidence to suggest that fasting women have a better response to endurance training than weight training,[36] while men may fare better with weights. Anecdotally, men tend to find working out on an empty stomach easier to accomplish than women.

In terms of general health, the benefits of occasional, short-term fasting for both sexes are pretty clear. Although quite a few human studies have been done with male volunteers, others have been done with a mixed group or mainly female volunteers. Those in Dr. Krista Varady's studies have been almost all women; Dr. Michelle Harvie's volunteers, all women. Their results are striking and positive, though further trials are required to analyze the precise effects of fasting on hormones, particularly among women of different ages. As with all recommendations in this book, be cautious and self-aware. Fasting is not meant to be a struggle; it's intended as a well-marked route to good health. If, for whatever reason, short bouts of fasting interrupt your menstrual cycle or your sleep pattern, modify your approach till you find a comfortable balance that works for you.

Can I fast if I'm trying to get pregnant?

Do not fast. Period. The science is still unfolding, and we simply don't have enough clinical trials to assess the total effects of limited fasting on fertility; always, therefore, err on the side of caution. Do not fast if you are already pregnant. Fasting is also absolutely forbidden for children; they are still growing and should not be subjected to nutritional stress of any type. Similarly, if you have an underlying medical condition, visit your primary care physician, as you would before embarking on any weight-loss regimen.

Who else shouldn't fast?

If you are in reasonable health, short fasts (including, don't forget, the 500- or 600-calorie allowance on the fast day) should be fine. If you are on medication of any description, please see your doctor first. There are certain groups for whom fasting is not advised. Type 1 diabetics are included in this list, along with anyone suffering from an eating disorder. If you are already extremely lean, do not fast. Children should never fast, so this is a plan for over-eighteens only.

Will I get headaches?

If you do, it may be due to dehydration rather than a lack of calories. You might experience mild withdrawal symptoms from sugar (or caffeine, if you've dropped it), but the brevity of your fast shouldn't make this of special concern. Keep drinking water. Treat a headache as you otherwise would;

if fasting today is making you feel particularly unwell, stop. You are in charge.

Should I worry about low blood sugar?

If you are in reasonably good health, your body is a remarkably efficient and functional machine, capable of—in fact, designed for—the effective regulation of blood sugar. Short-term fasting is unlikely to yield a hypoglycemic response. The recently propagated idea that we need to graze to avoid a "blood sugar crash" is a myth; if you follow the guidelines set out here and eat low-GI foods on a fast day, your blood glucose should remain stable. But don't overdo it. If you fast for extended periods, longer than the biweekly, twenty-four-hour modified eating program recommended here, you may experience a drop in blood pressure, a drop in glucose levels, and feelings of dizziness. So fast smart. If you are a type 2 diabetic, consult your doctor before embarking on *any* dietary change.

Will I feel tired?

The Illinois researchers hypothesized that subjects would feel "less energetic on fast days, and would therefore be less physically active."[37] They found no such thing, suggesting that short-term, deliberate, modified fasting will not leave you beat. As in normal life, you'll undoubtedly have up days and down days, good days and bad. Anecdotally, many intermittent fasters we have encountered report a boost to energy rather than a depletion. See how you fare. You may find that a fast day ends sooner than most—an early night, no alcohol, and plentiful sleep being a great way to arrive at breakfast sooner.

But will I go to bed hungry?

Probably not, though it will depend on your particular metabolism, and how you timed your fast-day calorie consumption. If you feel hungry, take your mind off it—a bubble bath, a good book, a stretch out, a cup of herbal tea. Get psychology on your side: congratulate yourself on reaching the end of another fast day. Surprisingly perhaps, fasters report that they don't wake up ravenous and run for the fridge as soon as the alarm goes off. Hunger is a subtle beast, and your appetite will soon find its rhythm.

Surprisingly perhaps, fasters report that they don't wake up ravenous and run for the fridge as soon as the alarm goes off. Hunger is a subtle beast, and your appetite will soon find its rhythm.

A MONTH OF 500-CALORIE MEALS

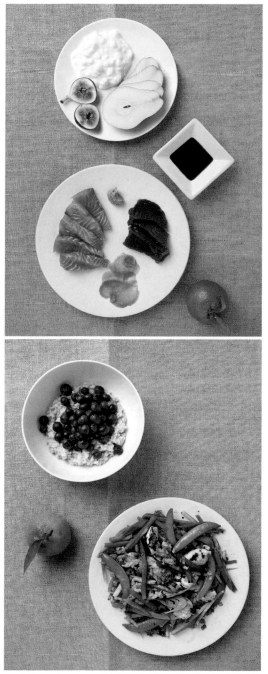

Breakfast: Cottage cheese, sliced pear, and a fresh fig.

142 calories

(See page 130.)

Dinner: Salmon and tuna sashimi with soy sauce, wasabi, pickled ginger, and a tangerine.

352 calories

(See page 130.)

Total calorie count: 494

Breakfast: Oatmeal with fresh blueberries.

190 calories

(See page 131.)

Dinner: Chicken stir-fry and a tangerine.

306 calories

(See page 131.)

Total calorie count: 496

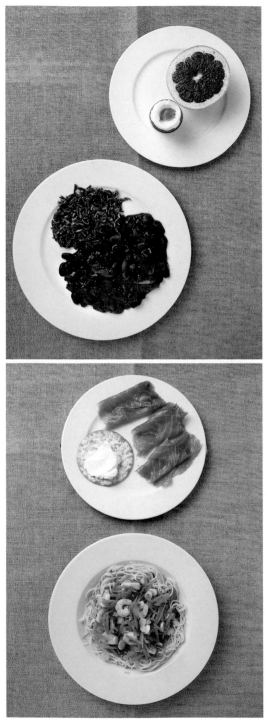

Breakfast: Boiled egg and half a grapefruit.

125 calories

(See page 132.)

Dinner: Vegetarian chili with brown rice.

371 calories

(See page 132.)

Total calorie count: 496

Breakfast: Smoked salmon and a cracker spread with low-fat whipped cream cheese.

178 calories

(See page 132.)

Dinner: Thai salad.

322 calories

(See page 133.)

Total calorie count: 500

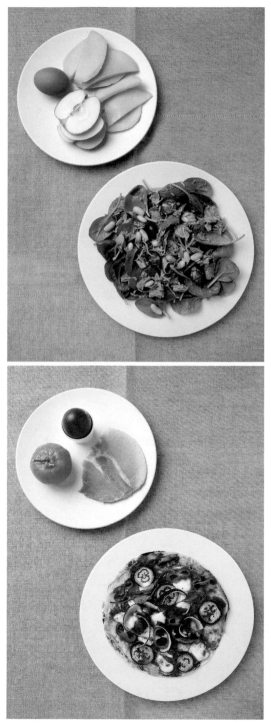

Breakfast: Sliced apple, mango, and a boiled egg.

223 calories

(See page 134.)

Dinner: Tuna, bean, and garlic salad. Dressing: crushed garlic, lemon zest and juice, and white wine vinegar.

267 calories

(See page 134.)

Total calorie count: 490

Breakfast: Boiled egg, a slice of ham, and a tangerine.

140 calories

(See page 135.)

Dinner: Vegetarian pizza.

358 calories

(See page 135.)

Total calorie count: 498

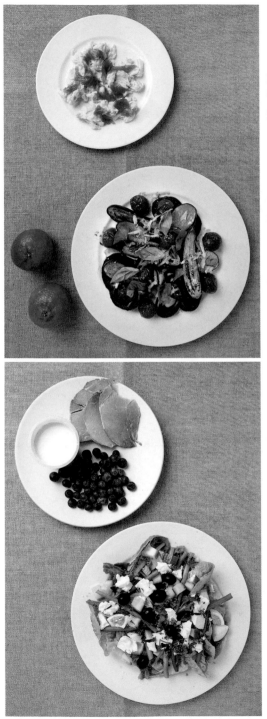

Breakfast: Smoked salmon scramble.

256 calories

(See page 136.)

Dinner: Roasted vegetables and two tangerines.

244 calories

(See page 136.)

Total calorie count: 500

Breakfast: Yogurt with blueberries and six slices of ham.

130 calories

(See page 137.)

Dinner: Feta niçoise salad.

360 calories

(See page 137.)

Total calorie count: 490

A MONTH OF 600-CALORIE MEALS

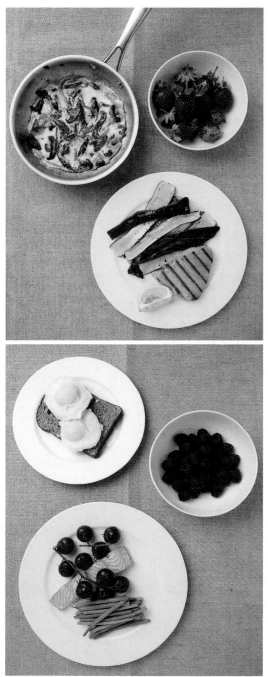

Breakfast: Mushroom and spinach frittata and a bowl of strawberries.

283 calories

(See page 139.)

Dinner: Seared tuna with grilled vegetables.

312 calories

(See page 139.)

Total calorie count: 595

Breakfast: Two poached eggs on a slice of whole-grain toast and a bowl of raspberries.

288 calories

(See page 140.)

Dinner: Roasted salmon with cherry tomatoes and green beans.

304 calories

(See page 140.)

Total calorie count: 592

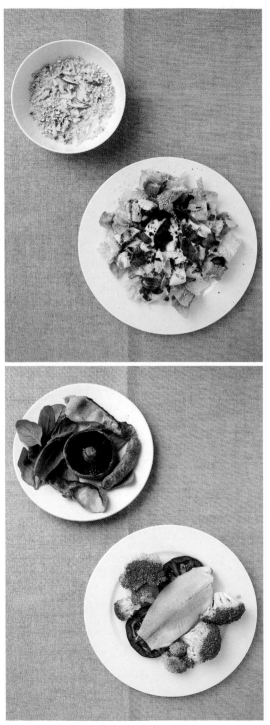

Breakfast: Muesli with grated apple.

308 calories

(See page 141.)

Dinner: No-carb Caesar salad.

292 calories

(See page 141.)

Total calorie count: 600

Breakfast: Modified English breakfast.

177 calories

(See page 143.)

Dinner: Mackerel and tomatoes *en papillote* with broccoli florets.

415 calories

(See page 143.)

Total calorie count: 592

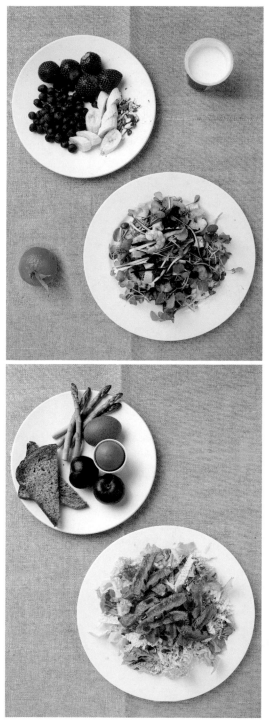

Breakfast: Yogurt, sliced banana, strawberries, blueberries, and almonds.

279 calories

(See page 144.)

Dinner: Shrimp, watercress, and avocado salad and a tangerine.

320 calories

(See page 144.)

Total calorie count: 599

Breakfast: Boiled eggs, asparagus spears, whole-grain toast, and two plums.

331 calories

(See page 146.)

Dinner: Thai steak salad.

260 calories

(See page 146.)

Total calorie count: 591

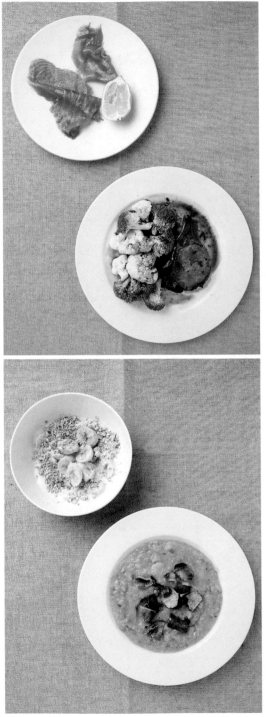

Breakfast: Smoked salmon and lemon wedges.

199 calories

(See page 147.)

Dinner: Roast pork with cauliflower and broccoli.

396 calories

(See page 147.)

Total calorie count: 595

Breakfast: Yogurt with sliced banana and muesli.

205 calories

(See page 147.)

Dinner: Bacon and butterbean soup.

386 calories

(See page 147.)

Total calorie count: 591

Will my body go into "starvation mode" and hang on to fat?

Since you're not restricting calories every day, your body will not enter the fabled "starvation mode." Your fasting will never be intense. It will only ever be conservative and short-lived, so while your body will burn energy from its fat stores, it will not consume muscle tissue. Research has shown that occasional fasting does not suppress the metabolism.[38] Even extreme fasting—an absolute fast for three consecutive days[39] or on every other day for three weeks[40]—generates no decrease in basal metabolic rate. Nor does intermittent fasting raise levels of the hunger-stimulating hormone ghrelin. Researchers at Pennington Biomedical Research Center in Louisiana found that "ghrelin was unchanged in both the men and the women, even after 36 hours of fasting."[41] If you follow the moderate, judicious approach advised here, a short window without food is a scientifically sanctioned path to health and well-being.

What if everyone around me is eating on one of my fast days?

Participate, but with a nonchalant awareness. While support from family and friends is an asset, making a song and dance about your fast will only cause you to feel self-conscious, turning the diet into an obstruction, a hurdle, rather than something that should slot happily and calmly into your life. Remember your trump card: you'll eat normally again tomorrow. Some days, of course, are tougher than others. As Dr. Varady noted among her trial subjects, hunger spiked at week eight: "We speculate that this may have occurred because this study week corresponded to Memorial Day weekend, and subjects may have felt hungrier while attending food-related celebrations."[42]

If you know that you have a social event or a food-related celebration on your schedule, fast the day before or the day after. The flexibility of the plan explicitly means—in fact, it demands—that you still go to that wedding, birthday, anniversary dinner, christening, bar mitzvah, supper date, posh restaurant. Take a break for Christmas, Easter, Thanksgiving, Diwali. Yes, you may well put on a little weight, but this is a life, not a life sentence. You can always deviate, eat chips and dips and things on sticks, and then revert to more challenging fasting once the party's over.

What if I'm currently obese?

Clinical trials have concluded that intermittent fasting is a sustainable—indeed, one of the most effective—ways for obese individuals to lose weight and keep it off; the larger you are, the greater your initial weight loss is likely to be. If you are obese, it's likely that for whatever reasons, traditional restrictive diets have failed for you. The FastDiet is different because of its flexibility, its war on guilt, and its allowing of "pleasure foods" on nonfast days. The Illinois studies have shown that obese people were able to quickly adapt to alternate-day modified fasting. They were also able to maintain physical activity despite fasting. In conclusion, "overweight and obese patients appear to experience significant improvements with IF regimes."[43] As with any underlying medical condition, we recommend that you fast under supervision.

Should I add a third day if I want to see accelerated results?

There's no reason not to; that is, after all, what Dr. Krista Varady's ADFs (alternate-day fasters) effectively do. However, beware of "fast fatigue." One of the keys to its success is that the FastDiet requires only short-lived dedication. Ask your body to do more than that and it may revolt and refuse to behave, making the recommended fasting program harder to achieve. Experience tells us that two days is enough. If, however, you have a date and a small size of party pants on standby, an occasional, single sneaky extra day shouldn't hurt. Don't, however, try a lengthy crash diet. Unless you are obese and it is medically supervised, it just isn't worth it.

I'm already slim enough, but would like to enjoy the health benefits of intermittent fasting. Is that possible?

If you are already at a reasonable, happy weight, you can still fast effectively, but consider adapting your consumption on nonfast days to encompass more calorie-dense foods. The main researchers we talked to in this field are all slim and they still fast. With practice, you will discover an amicable balance between fasting and feeding that keeps your weight in the prescribed range. Alternatively, fast once every eight to ten days rather than twice a week. There have been no studies to illuminate the effects of doing this, but use your common sense and watch the scale; don't slide. If, however, you are already extremely lean or suffering from an eating disorder, fasting of any description is not advised. If in doubt, see your doctor.

The FastDiet is likely to prolong your life. It will moderate your appetite and help you lose weight. Its effects are quickly felt, often within a week of starting your simple biweekly mini fasts.

Is it too late to start?

On the contrary, there's no time to lose. The FastDiet is likely to prolong your life. It will moderate your appetite and help you lose weight. Its effects are quickly felt, often within a week of starting your simple biweekly mini fasts. It all points to a healthier, leaner, longer old age, fewer doctors' appointments, more energy, greater resistance to disease. Our advice? Start yesterday.

How long should I continue?

Interestingly, the FastDiet's on/off eating scheme looks a lot like the approach of many naturally slim people. Some days they'll pick, other days, they'll tuck into treats. In the long run, this is how the FastDiet goes. As you settle into the routine, you'll naturally moderate your calorie intake on fast days and feed days, until the process is innate. When you reach your target weight, you can change the frequency of your fast. Play with it. But don't drift; stay alert. Your aim is a permanent life change, not a blip, not a fad, not a dinner-party chat. This is a long-distance route to sustained weight loss. Accept that it is something you will do, in a form that suits you, indefinitely. For as long as life.

The future of fasting: where next?

Fasting, as we mentioned at the beginning, has been practiced for many thousands of years and yet science is only just starting to catch up. The first evidence of the long-term benefits of calorie restriction were found just over eighty years ago, when nutritionists working with rats at Cornell University discovered that if you severely restrict the amount they eat, they live longer. Much longer.

Since then, the evidence has continued to mount that animals not only live longer, healthier lives if they are calorie restricted, but that they also do so if they are intermittently fasted. In recent years the research has moved on from rodents to humans, and we are seeing the same patterns of improvement.

So where do we go from here? Dr. Valter Longo, who has done so much pioneering work with IGF-1, is running a number of human trials in conjunction with colleagues at the University of Southern California, looking at the impact of fasting on cancer. They have already demonstrated that fasting will cut your risk of developing cancer; now they want to see if fasting will also improve the efficacy of chemotherapy and radiotherapy.

Dr. Krista Varady of the University of Illinois at Chicago has a number of projects planned. She has a trial running at the moment looking at how well people are able to tolerate alternate-day fasting in the long run. This is critical research because the success or failure of a dietary intervention depends entirely on compliance. Will people stay on it? Last time we spoke, she was also bubbling with ideas for the future, including investigations into why people on ADF lose fat but don't seem to lose significant muscle mass, and why people on ADF don't seem to fully compensate for the calories they've missed by eating more on their feed days. She has many theories but needs more cold hard facts.

Dr. Mark Mattson of the National Institute on Aging is

adding all the time to the dozens of research papers he has already published on the effects of fasting, and intermittent fasting, on the brain. We are particularly interested to see the outcome of some of his current studies, which include looking further into what happens to the brains of human volunteers when put on an intermittent fasting regimen.

In addition, his team is looking at drug therapies, as they know that despite the benefits, many people may not want to fast. So they are, for example, looking into a drug called Byetta, used for the treatment of diabetes, but which also seems to activate the production of BDNF (brain-derived neurotrophic factor). This, in turn, as we've seen, seems to protect the brain against the ravages of aging. The hope is that Byetta or a related drug will, if not prevent dementia, at least slow its progression significantly.

Intermittent fasting has, until now, been one of the best-kept secrets in science. We look forward with a great deal of personal interest to seeing how this particular story unfolds.

CHAPTER THREE

Menu Plans

Fast Day Cooking Tips

1. Feel free to top up the low-calorie, low-GI leafy vegetables beyond the quantities given here. It is difficult to overdo it on leafy veggies, and if you need bulk, here's where you should get it. Roasted vegetables are tasty; lightly steamed is best. Invest in a tiered bamboo steamer, and cook your proteins and veggies in several health-packed, eco-friendly levels.

2. Some vegetables benefit from cooking; others are better eaten raw (see page 105 for more details). Cooking certain vegetables—including carrots, spinach, mushrooms, asparagus, cabbage, and peppers—breaks down the cell structure without

destroying vitamins, allowing you to absorb more goodies. For raw vegetables, a mandoline makes preparation easy and swift.

3. Fast days should be low-fat rather than no-fat. A teaspoon of olive oil can be used in cooking, or drizzled over vegetables for flavor, or use an olive oil spray to get a thin film. And nuts and fattier meats such as pork are included in the plans. Do include a light oil dressing on your salads; it means that you are more likely to absorb their fat-soluble vitamins.

4. The acid in lemon or orange dressings means that you will absorb more iron from leafy greens such as spinach and kale. Watercress with orange is a great combination, perhaps scattered with some sesame and sunflower seeds or blanched almonds for a little protein and crunch.

5. Always cook in a nonstick pan to cut down on calorie-dense fats. Add a splash of water rather than more oil if the food sticks to the pan.

6. Weigh your food *after* preparing it (trimming, slicing, chopping, and so on) so that the calorie count is correct. You will need to invest in a kitchen scale.

7. Dairy is also included here: choose lower-fat cheeses and 1% or 2% milk; avoid full-fat yogurt in favor of

low-fat alternatives. Drop the lattes and toss out the butter on a fast day—they are calorie traps.

8. Similarly, avoid starchy white carbohydrates (bread, potatoes, pasta) and opt instead for low-GI carbs such as vegetables, beans and lentils, and slow-burn whole-grain cereals. Choose brown rice and quinoa. Oatmeal for breakfast will keep you fuller for longer than cold cereal.

9. Ensure that you get some fiber in your fast: eat the skin of apples and pears, have oats for breakfast, keep those leafy vegetables coming in.

10. Add flavor where you can: chili flakes will give a kick to any savory dish. Vinegars, including balsamic, will lend acidity. Add fresh herbs, too— they are virtually calorie free but give personality to a plate.

11. Eating protein will help keep you fuller longer. Stick to low-fat proteins, including nuts and beans. Remove the skin and fat from meats before cooking.

> Eating protein will help keep you fuller longer.

12. Soup can be a savior on a fast day, particularly if you choose a light broth packed with

THE FASTDIET

leafy vegetables (miso soup would be ideal). Soup is satiating, and a good way of using up ingredients languishing in the fridge.

13. Use agave as a sweetener if required; it's low-GI.

500-Calories-a-Day Menus

Day 1

Breakfast (142 calories)
   Scant ½ cup low-fat cottage cheese (78 calories)
   1 sliced pear (40 calories)
   1 fresh fig (24 calories)

Dinner (352 calories)
   SASHIMI (327 calories)
   3 to 5 pieces each of salmon (3.5 ounces/180 calories)
      and tuna sashimi (3.5 ounces/136 calories)
   2 teaspoons soy sauce (2 calories)
   Wasabi
   Pickled ginger (9 calories)

   1 tangerine (25 calories)

Daily Total: 494

Day 2

Breakfast (190 calories)

Oatmeal made with 1.4 ounces steel-cut oats (160 calories) and water

Scant ½ cup fresh blueberries (30 calories)

Dinner (306 calories)

CHICKEN STIR-FRY (281 calories)

Cut a 5-ounce chicken breast fillet (148 calories) into strips. Stir-fry in a nonstick skillet in 1 teaspoon olive oil (27 calories) with 1 teaspoon finely chopped ginger (2 calories), 1 tablespoon chopped cilantro (3 calories), 1 clove garlic, crushed (3 calories), 2 teaspoons soy sauce (3 calories), and the juice of ½ lemon (1 calorie) until the chicken is lightly browned. Add water if it sticks.

Add ½ cup trimmed snow peas (12 calories), 1½ cups shredded cabbage (26 calories), and 2 large carrots, peeled and cut into thin strips (56 calories). Stir-fry for 5 to 10 minutes more, until the chicken is cooked through. Add water if necessary.

1 tangerine (25 calories)

Daily Total: 496

Day 3

Breakfast (125 calories)

1 small boiled egg (90 calories)

½ grapefruit (35 calories)

Dinner (371 calories)

VEGETARIAN CHILI (258 calories)

Fry 1 clove garlic, chopped (3 calories), and ½ large fresh red chile, seeded and finely chopped (3 calories), in 1 teaspoon olive oil (27 calories) in a nonstick skillet. Add a pinch of ground cumin and 2 small white mushrooms or 1 large white mushroom, chopped (3 calories). Cook for 5 minutes, adding water if it sticks.

Stir in ½ of a 14-ounce can chopped tomatoes with juices (32 calories) and scant ½ of a 14-ounce can kidney beans, rinsed and drained (190 calories). Simmer for 10 minutes.

Serve with ½ cup cooked brown rice (113 calories).

Daily Total: 496

Day 4

Breakfast (178 calories)

4 ounces smoked salmon (132 calories)

1 plain Ryvita cracker (35 calories)

1½ teaspoons low-fat whipped cream cheese (11 calories)

Dinner (322 calories)

THAI SALAD (322 calories)

Soak 1.8 ounces rice vermicelli noodles (194 calories) in water according to package instructions.

Combine 2 tablespoons Thai fish sauce (20 calories), the juice of 1 lime (1 calorie), 1 teaspoon sugar (16 calories), 2 scallions (white and green parts), trimmed and thinly sliced (5 calories), and 1 very small red chile, finely chopped (1 calorie) in a bowl. Mix well. Add 10 very small cooked and peeled shrimp (30 calories) and 2 large carrots, peeled and grated (55 calories). Drain the noodles and add. Toss well.

Daily Total: 500 calories

Day 5

Breakfast (171 calories)

STRAWBERRY SMOOTHIE (171 calories)

Blend 1 small banana (95 calories), a generous ½ cup fat-free plain yogurt (62 calories), 7 strawberries (1-inch diameter), trimmed and hulled (14 calories), a splash of water, and some cracked ice until thick and creamy. Serve immediately.

Dinner (325 calories)

OVEN-BAKED TILAPIA (202 calories)

Preheat the oven or a toaster oven to 400°F. Very lightly coat a small baking dish with cooking spray. Place a 7- to 8-ounce tilapia fillet (202 calories) in the dish and sprinkle with your favorite dried herbs or ground spices. Bake for 15 to 20 minutes, until cooked through.

Serve with a small poached egg (90 calories) and ⅔ cup lightly steamed broccoli florets or chopped broccoli rabe (33 calories).

Daily Total: 496 calories

Day 6

Breakfast (223 calories)

1 small apple, sliced (47 calories)

1 small mango, peeled and pitted (86 calories)

1 small boiled egg (90 calories)

Dinner (267 calories)

TUNA, BEAN, AND GARLIC SALAD (267 calories)

Combine 1½ cups canned cannellini beans, drained and rinsed (108 calories), one 5-ounce can solid white tuna in spring water, drained (119 calories), 2 ounces grape tomatoes (16 calories), and 1 loosely packed cup baby spinach (8 calories) in a salad bowl.

In a small bowl, combine 1 clove garlic, crushed (3 calories), the juice and grated zest of lemon (1 calorie), ½ teaspoon olive oil (12 calories), and a splash of white wine vinegar. Drizzle over the salad and toss to mix well.

Daily Total: 490 calories

Day 7

Breakfast (140 calories)

1 small boiled egg (90 calories)

3 ultra-thin slices 97% fat-free ham (25 calories)

1 tangerine (25 calories)

Dinner (358 calories)

VEGETABLE PIZZA (358 calories)

Preheat the oven or a toaster oven to 400°F. Top one 8-inch whole-wheat tortilla (144 calories) with 1 tablespoon tomato puree (5 calories) and 2 ounces fresh mozzarella cheese, diced (159 calories). Scatter with about 6 ounces chopped lightly steamed vegetables (50 calories); mushrooms, red pepper, zucchini, red onion, eggplant, spinach are all okay. Sprinkle with Italian herb seasoning. Bake for 5 to 10 minutes, until the cheese has melted.

Daily Total: 498 calories

Day 8

Breakfast (256 calories)

SMOKED SALMON SCRAMBLE (256 calories)

Whisk together 2 small eggs (180 calories) and 1 table-spoon skim milk (5 calories). Scramble in a dry nonstick skillet until cooked but not completely dry. Remove from the heat and stir in 1.8 ounces smoked salmon, cut in slivers (71 calories).

Dinner (244 calories)

ROASTED VEGETABLES WITH BALSAMIC VINEGAR AND PARMESAN (195 calories)

Preheat the oven or a toaster oven to 400°F. Very lightly coat a baking dish with cooking spray. In the baking dish, combine 10 cherry tomatoes (27 calories), ½ small zucchini, trimmed and sliced (9 calories), ½ cup cubed eggplant (11 calories), and 1 scant cup sliced red bell pepper (50 calories). Scatter with fresh basil leaves (1 calorie) and drizzle with ½ teaspoon balsamic vinegar (6 calories). Bake for 20 to 25 minutes, stirring occasionally, until the vegetables are softened and lightly browned. Sprinkle with ¼ cup grated Parmesan cheese (90 calories) before serving.

2 tangerines (50 calories)

Daily Total: 500 calories

Day 9

Breakfast (130 calories)

Generous ½ cup fat-free plain yogurt (62 calories)

¼ cup fresh blueberries (18 calories)

6 ultra-thin slices 97% fat-free ham (50 calories)

Dinner (360 calories)

FETA NIÇOISE SALAD (360 calories)

Hard-cook, cool, peel, and chop 1 small egg (90 calories). In a salad bowl, combine the egg with 1 medium leaf romaine lettuce, chopped (3 calories), ¼ cup chopped steamed green beans (12 calories), and 1 scant cup chopped unpeeled cucumber (10 calories). Toss to combine.

Top with scant ⅔ cup crumbled feta cheese (225 calories), 1½ sliced pitted super colossal black olives (19 calories), and 1 tablespoon chopped parsley (1 calorie). Drizzle with white wine vinegar and serve.

Daily Total: 490 calories

Day 10

Breakfast (290 calories)

CHEESE AND TOMATO OMELET (290 calories)

Whisk together 2 small eggs (180 calories) and 1 tablespoon skim milk (5 calories). Cook undisturbed in a dry nonstick skillet until set but still slightly moist on top. Top with 2 very thin slices fresh tomato (5 calories) and 1 slice American cheese (100 calories). Remove from the heat, cover, and let sit until the cheese has melted.

Dinner (209 calories)

FAST-DAY INSALATA CAPRESE (191 calories)

Slice 2 ounces fresh mozzarella cheese (159 calories). Slice 1 medium beefsteak tomato (26 calories). Alternate the slices on a plate. Scatter with fresh basil leaves and drizzle with ½ teaspoon balsamic vinegar (6 calories).

Scant ½ cup strawberries, trimmed and hulled (18 calories)

Daily Total: 499 calories

600-Calories-a-Day Menus

Day 1

Breakfast (283 calories)

MUSHROOM AND SPINACH FRITTATA (245 calories)

Fry ½ medium onion, sliced (27 calories), in 1 teaspoon olive oil (27 calories) in a nonstick skillet until translucent. Add 2 small white mushrooms or 1 large white mushroom, chopped (3 calories), and cook until the mushrooms are barely tender. Add 1 loosely packed cup baby spinach (8 calories) and cook for 2 minutes more. Pour in 2 small eggs, beaten (180 calories). Cook undisturbed for 5 minutes, and finish under a hot broiler until the eggs are set.

1 scant cup whole strawberries (38 calories)

Dinner (312 calories)

SEARED TUNA WITH GRILLED VEGETABLES (312 calories)

Cut 1 small red bell pepper, stemmed and seeded (38 calories), and 1 small zucchini, trimmed (18 calories), into slices about ¼-inch wide. Toss in a bowl with 1 teaspoon olive oil (27 calories). Season lightly. Heat a grill pan over medium-high heat and grill the vegetables 5 minutes per side, flipping the slices once. Serve on a plate and dress with a squeeze of lemon.

In the same pan, grill a 7-ounce tuna steak (229 calories), flipping once, until done to your taste. Plate with the vegetables, with another squeeze of lemon.

Daily Total: 595 calories

Day 2

Breakfast (288 calories)
    2 small poached eggs (180 calories)
    1 slice whole-grain toast (78 calories)
    30 fresh raspberries (30 calories)

Dinner (304 calories)
    ROASTED SALMON WITH TOMATOES (279 calories)
    Preheat the oven or a toaster oven to 400°F. Very lightly coat a small baking dish with cooking spray. In the dish, place a 5-ounce skinless salmon fillet (252 calories) with 10 cherry tomatoes (27 calories). Bake for 15 to 20 minutes, until the fish is cooked.
    Serve with ½ cup sliced steamed green beans (25 calories).

Daily Total: 592 calories

Day 3

Breakfast (308 calories)

BREAKFAST MUESLI (308 calories)

Mix ⅔ cup old-fashioned rolled oats (201 calories) with 1 small apple, grated, including skin (47 calories). Stir in ⅔ cup skim milk (60 calories). Let soak briefly to soften.

Dinner (292 calories)

NO-CARB CAESAR SALAD (292 calories)

Heat a grill pan over medium-high heat. Grill 2 slices Canadian bacon (86 calories) for 4 to 5 minutes, flipping once. Set aside to cool, then coarsely chop.

Cut a 5-ounce chicken breast fillet (148 calories) in half to make two thinner fillets. Grill for 3 to 4 minutes on each side, until cooked through. Cut into cubes. Place the chicken on a bed of about 2 cups chopped romaine lettuce (16 calories). Sprinkle with 1 tablespoon grated Parmesan cheese (22 calories) and drizzle with 1 tablespoon fat-free Caesar salad dressing (20 calories). Sprinkle the bacon over the top.

Daily Total: 600 calories

Day 4

Breakfast (340 calories)

CHEESE AND TOMATO OMELET (290 calories)

Whisk together 2 small eggs (180 calories) and 1 table-spoon skim milk (5 calories). Cook undisturbed in a dry nonstick skillet until set but still slightly moist on top. Top with 2 very thin slices fresh tomato (5 calories) and 1 slice American cheese (100 calories). Remove from the heat, cover, and let sit until the cheese has melted.

2 tangerines (50 calories)

Dinner (260 calories)

MARINATED STEAK AND ASIAN CABBAGE SALAD
(260 calories)

Marinate a 3-ounce piece sirloin steak (120 calories) in a mixture of 1 teaspoon soy sauce (1 calorie), juice of 1 lime (2 calories) and 1 clove garlic, crushed (3 calories), for about 10 minutes. Heat a grill pan over medium-high heat. Remove steak from marinade and grill to desired doneness, turning once. Set aside to cool.

For the Asian cabbage salad: in a bowl, combine 1 small carrot, peeled and grated (18 calories), 1½ cups shredded savoy cabbage (24 calories), and a handful of cilantro sprigs, chopped (1 calorie). In a separate bowl, combine 1 teaspoon sugar (16 calories) with 1 tablespoon Thai fish sauce (10 calories), juice of 1 lime (2 calories), and 1 clove garlic, crushed (3 calories). Pour over the salad and toss to combine. Arrange on plate. Slice steak and arrange on salad. Top with 1 tablespoon chopped unsalted dry-roasted peanuts (60 calories).

Daily Total: 600 calories

Day 5

Breakfast (177 calories)

MODIFIED ENGLISH BREAKFAST (177 calories)
Cook 1½ strips thick-sliced bacon (107 calories) until crisp. Heat 1 small brown 'n' serve sausage (59 calories). Grill 1 small portobello mushroom cap (3 calories). Arrange on top of 1 loosely packed cup baby spinach (8 calories).

Dinner (415 calories)

MACKEREL AND TOMATOES EN PAPILLOTE (381 calories)
Preheat the oven or a toaster oven to 400°F. Lay out a square of foil and very lightly coat it with cooking oil spray. Arrange 2 medium-large tomatoes, sliced (30 calories), on the foil and top with a 6-ounce mackerel fillet (351 calories). Bring two opposite corners of the foil together and fold over tightly. Repeat with the other corners to make a tight packet. Roast for 10 to 15 minutes, or until fish is cooked through. Place the packet on a plate and open carefully.

Serve with ⅔ cup lightly steamed broccoli florets or

chopped broccoli rabe (33 calories), dressed with juice of ½ lemon (1 calorie) and a light sprinkle of salt.

Daily Total: 592 calories

Day 6

Breakfast (279 calories)
Generous ½ cup fat-free plain yogurt (62 calories)
1 small banana, sliced (80 calories)
5 large strawberries (20 calories)
⅓ cup blueberries (25 calories)
6 almonds, chopped (92 calories)

Dinner (320 calories)
SHRIMP, WATERCRESS, AND AVOCADO SALAD (295 calories)
In a salad bowl, combine 1½ cups chopped watercress (6 calories) with 5 ounces peeled cooked shrimp (139 calories), ½ avocado, pitted, peeled, and diced (137 calories), 3 tablespoons finely chopped red onion (11 calories), and 1 tablespoon capers, drained and rinsed (2 calories). Sprinkle with white wine vinegar and toss.

1 tangerine (25 calories)

Daily Total: 599 calories

Day 7

Breakfast (261 calories)

HAM AND EGG BREAKFAST (261 calories)
Whisk together 2 small eggs (180 calories) and 1 table-spoon skim milk (5 calories). Scramble in a dry nonstick skillet until cooked to your desired doneness. Serve with 2.5 ounces 97% fat-free sliced ham (76 calories).

Dinner (333 calories)

SPICED DAL (213 calories)
Fry 1 small onion, thinly sliced (22 calories), 1 clove garlic, crushed (3 calories), and 1 teaspoon finely chopped ginger (2 calories) in 1 teaspoon olive oil (27 calories) in a small saucepan for 5 minutes, until the onion is translucent. Add 1 cup water, ¼ cup red lentils, picked over and rinsed (159 calories), and a pinch each of ground cumin, ground coriander, ground turmeric, cayenne pepper, salt, and pepper. Bring to a boil, lower the heat to medium-low, and simmer for 20 minutes, or until the lentils are tender.

Garnish with ⅓ cup fat-free plain yogurt (40 calories) and serve with 1 pappadum (Indian lentil cracker, available in the international aisle) (80 calories).

Daily Total: 594 calories

Day 8

Breakfast (331 calories)

    2 small soft-boiled eggs (180 calories)

    5 lightly steamed asparagus spears (33 calories), to dip

    1 slice whole-grain toast (78 calories)

    2 small plums (40 calories)

Dinner (260 calories)

THAI STEAK SALAD (260 calories)

Grill a 5-ounce sirloin steak (188 calories) until cooked to your preferred doneness. Set aside to cool to room temperature. Slice the steak very thin across the grain.

In a bowl, combine 2 cups shredded romaine lettuce (16 calories) and 1 cup shredded savoy cabbage (24 calories). In a separate bowl, combine the juice of 1 lime (2 calories), 1 teaspoon sugar (16 calories), 1 clove garlic, crushed (3 calories), 1 very small red chile, seeded and finely chopped (1 calorie), and 1 tablespoon Thai fish sauce (10 calories). Pour over the salad and toss to combine. Place the salad on a plate and arrange the steak slices on top.

Daily Total: 591 calories

Day 9

Breakfast (199 calories)

6 ounces smoked salmon (198 calories)

½ lemon, cut into wedges (1 calorie)

Dinner (396 calories)

4.5 ounces sliced lean roast pork loin (302 calories)

1 tablespoon defatted pan juices (60 calories)

Generous ½ cup steamed cauliflower florets (17 calories)

⅓ cup steamed chopped broccoli (17 calories)

Daily Total: 595 calories

Day 10

Breakfast (205 calories)

Generous ½ cup fat-free plain yogurt (62 calories)

1 small banana, sliced (95 calories)

2 tablespoons sugar-free plain muesli, *not* granola (48 calories)

Dinner (386 calories)

BACON & BUTTERBEAN SOUP (386 calories)

Fry 2 strips bacon, chopped (116 calories) in 1 teaspoon olive oil (27 calories) in a saucepan for 2 minutes, until the fat starts to render out. Add ½ small onion, finely chopped (11 calories), 3 tablespoons chopped leek

(11 calories), ½ carrot, peeled and thinly sliced (14 calories), and 1 stalk celery, chopped (1 calorie). Cook for 5 minutes, until the onions are translucent, adding a splash of water if it sticks. Add ½ a 14-ounce can butterbeans or lima beans, drained and rinsed (206 calories) and 1 cup water. Bring to a boil, then lower the heat and simmer for 20 minutes, until the beans are very soft. Season to taste.

Transfer the mixture to a blender and puree until the desired consistency, or mash with a potato masher for a chunkier texture.

Daily Total: 591 calories

Case Studies

Dear Dr. Mosley,

My partner and I both decided this made a lot of sense and have been following your 5:2 regimen since the program aired at the start of the month. So far we've lost three pounds each, although we weren't overweight before, and have still been able to poke in a few portions of curry and cake on feed days. We definitely plan to continue fasting in some form in the long term.

As an asthmatic over 40, I'm very interested in the putative effects on inflammation as well as all the other great antiaging protection . . . I also have a bit of chronic leg pain from a running injury and will be keen to see if it boosts muscle and nerve repair over the coming months. Basically I'm hoping my body will try to heal itself a bit better.

Thanks again for a great bit of science broadcasting.

Alison Rae

Hi,

I have been IF now for the last 14 weeks. I have lost [nearly] 9½ pounds, and 9½ inches. On previous diets I have never got below 140 pounds.

> Start weight 145.6 pounds
> Current weight 136.4 pounds
> Height 5'6"
> Inch loss:
>> Bust 1¼"
>> Midriff ½"
>> Waist 1¾"
>> Abdomen 2½"
>> Hips 2½"
>> Thighs ½" each leg
> Cholesterol has not changed since last test over
>> 1 year ago; reading is 4.9. Blood glucose also
>> no change. Reading 4.7
> Improvements other than weight loss:
>> Eyes look brighter and clearer
>> More energy
>> Sleeping better
>> Clearer head and better mental clarity (although
>>> not tested I feel that I can remember things
>>> more easily)
>> Feel healthy

Hope my feedback is useful.
Kind regards,

Sarah Humphries

Hi, Dr. Mosley,

OK, fast two of week 13 was completed yesterday and as promised, here's an update for 13 weeks/3 months/ 1 whole quarter of intermittent fasting.

The program involves eating only 600 calories on two selected, nonconsecutive days of the week. Apart from the two days a week, that's it. The rest of the time, I eat/ drink what I want. You don't need to exercise or count calories on a daily basis, you don't feel hungry 24/7 and, best of all, you don't die of starvation. Tonight is Indian night, tomorrow is steak night and Sunday is probably Italian. Every night is booze night. That doesn't sound like too onerous a regime to me. It's fair to say that my overall weekly calorie consumption (beyond just fast days) has reduced, not because I'm avoiding eating on the feed days, but purely because I'm just not as hungry.

Over the past 13 weeks, I've been developing the regime to suit myself and have got into a fairly settled Monday & Thursday routine. I consume nothing at all during the day apart from 3 or 4 teas/coffees (just marginally whitened) and about 1 to 1.5 liters of tap water. I come home and I do a 10-mile thrash on a cycle turbo trainer. Last night, I did it in 30 minutes & 25 seconds. To all intents and purposes, an average of 20 mph for 30 minutes. I've set up the trainer on the advice of some pretty serious chaps on the Fool's dedicated cycling forum. The idea is to try and make it "feel" as close to a road bike as possible. Using that assumption, my 10-miler burns around 550 calories. By doing it before you eat on a fast day, the theory (I guess) is that you're forcing your body to burn body fat, rather than the carbs it would normally turn to for a short burst of energy.

Hunger-wise, well it's okay. I eat late prior to a fast day and that definitely helps. I find having even a small breakfast actually triggers hunger for the rest of the day, so I avoid everything until late on, when I have around 450 calories—240 cals of flavored rice and the rest as vegetables. It's easily managed—you actually don't get more hungry throughout the day and it's easy to take your mind off it by doing something. You DO have to approach a fast day in the right mindset though. If you don't, you'll have a pretty hellish time. Do it right and it's really quite a doddle.

So, when I started the regime in mid-August, I was a fraction of a pound off 196 and on the last notch of my belt (I know that's not very scientific and I wish I'd taken more measurements when I started, but hey-ho).

This morning, I tipped the scale at 177 pounds and the 4th notch on my belt is quite comfortable (the third is a wee bit loose). 1 notch = just about a fraction over 1 inch. The goal without exercise would be a pound a week (given that a 4,000 weekly calorie restriction = roughly 1 pound of body fat). With the 1 hour of exercise a week, I accelerated it by almost 50 percent to 19 pounds in the same period.

I'm keeping going until Christmas, when I hope to go to a 5:1+1 (the +1 being an 800- or 900-calorie day). If that works, then I'll stay on that for the rest of my time.

I went for a cycle last Sunday after having a full breakfast and it was incredibly easy. Loads of speed, the hills were actually fun and, apart from the chilliness, it was extremely enjoyable. The benefit of being fitter and having a fuelled-up body I guess. LOADS of energy.

Other benefits: I have suffered from asthma since I was a child. It's nowhere near as bad as it was when I was a kid, but now it's practically disappeared. My "peak flow" reading has gone up by over 30 percent in the 13 weeks— probably as a result of the weight loss allowing me to exercise harder.

I have suffered from asthma since I was a child. It's nowhere near as bad as it was when I was a kid, but now it's practically disappeared.

A wee bit girly here, but I'd say my skin complexion has improved dramatically. No zits or blackheads—even the touch of dry skin on my elbows has gone.

All the best

David Norvell

Hi, Michael,

Both my partner and myself watched your program and thought it was very interesting, so we decided to start the

5:2 fasting on the following Monday. (Always good to start new things on a Monday, I find!) I have done liquid fasting in the past, for weeks, and really liked it. But then I put the weight back on again, I found. This seems to work better . . .

> Height: 5'4"
> Weight: 183 pounds

I'm not very FAT as such, but I do need to lose weight, especially my tummy/waist—the exact place where it's not good for you to be fat . . . I know! My aim is to get to 143 to 154 pounds. But at my age, it's not so easy to lose weight as it used to be when I was younger (according to my GP).

> 6 Aug: 183 pounds (Started the fasting)
> 8 Aug: 180½ pounds
> 9 Aug: 178¼ pounds
> 14 Aug: 178¼ pounds
> 18 Aug: 176 pounds
> 23 Aug: 176 pounds
> 27 Aug: 175 pounds
> 6 Sept: 175 pounds
> 13 Sept: 172¾ pounds
> 21 Sept: 173¾ pounds

We both love the intermittent fasting. As you can see, I have lost some weight and the only reason it has not gone quicker is the fact I have not done as much exercise as I set out to do originally. We will certainly continue and I will keep weighing myself to check the progress.

We also find it makes us want to eat less the adjacent days, too. We do our two days on Tuesdays and Wednesdays. Come Thursday morning, I feel so "light" and full of energy, I don't want to "spoil" it by eating too much even if it's my feeding day . . .

We have our main "fasting meal" in the evening, as it's the time we see each other at home after work, to settle down and talk over dinner. It's probably not ideal from a calorie-burning aspect, but it's more practical for us and suits us best.

A typical fasting day main meal:

> Corn on the cob as starter
> Salmon fillet with garlic, lemon, herbs, salt, and
>   pepper and a minimum amount of olive oil OR a
>   two-egg omelet with onion, garlic, parsley, sliced
>   mushrooms
> Salad: various green salad leaves, tomatoes, red
>   onion, herbs, maybe beets
> Drink: water

During the day, we eat a banana and an apple.

I'm really grateful for you making this program and have passed it on to friends and family who have taken it on, too.

Best regards,

Britt Warg

I'm a neurophysiology & pharmacology student, researching Parkinson's. I'm not giving medical advice, or trying to tell people how to fast/diet/whatever. Inspired by the *Horizon* program, I decided to "self-experiment" if you will. This has now blossomed into a project that will be run at my university what with that fancy scientific method, and all . . . I'm interested in data, neurodegenerative disorders and what steps I can take in my own lifestyle that will decrease my occurrences of breast cancer.

I myself am a two-time (and counting) breast cancer patient, so I'm rather interested in what impact (if any) fasting lifestyles could have on recurrence.

From [my] blog, *Schrokit's Corner*:

It's not a *diet*

So seven weeks into 5:2 (or 2:5 as I like to call it since I think of my weeks starting with fasting and then five days of EATING) and still going strong. I'm a little over 14 pounds down, with Mr. Schrokit not too far behind (he keeps calling his jeans "fat man trousers" since he needs to do up his belt a few extra notches inward . . .)

Because the overall difference in my appearance and "result" is so easy to see (though people keep asking me if I changed my hair, got new glasses etc., they can't seem to pin down the weight loss, but I'm getting compliments galore),

I'm getting compliments galore.

when I talk to people about fasting, they seem
VERY keen to give it a go. In fact, many of
Mr. Schrokit's colleagues are on this so-called diet
and finding it very eye-opening about their own
eating habits.

But it's not a diet. The best description I've heard
so far is from blog commenter Gordon. It's a *strategy*,
to quote him, and I can't think of a better word
for it.

Aside from eating a healthy *balanced* diet,
whatever all the trendy diet books tell you, weight
control is really about the *aggregate* amount
of calories you consume in the long run. I've
mentioned this before, but the thing that fasting
does seem to do is help one get back in touch with
actual appetite. For example, hungry versus bored,
or hungry v. tired, hungry v. craving, and most of
all, hungry versus thirsty all seem a bit more obvious
after fasting a couple of days.

Nicole Slavin

For me, fasting—600 calories twice a week—has changed
my attitude to food and drink. It has broken a cycle of
overindulgence which caused my weight to rise steadily
for 30 years. We are creatures of habit, and without
realizing it slip into patterns of behavior which are difficult
to change. But now something profound has happened:

I perceive things more clearly and there is something about this new state of mind which reminds me of how I felt in my 20s when I had a BMI of around 22. I no longer feel comfortable if I have eaten too much, and I feel more in control. The habit is being broken. I suspect I will be on this diet more or less for the rest of my life.

David Cleevely

The "FastDiet" looks like a wonderful way of optimizing our well-being, our longevity, and a great way to lose weight, too. As you say, it is so much more than "just a diet," it is really a whole lifestyle, and importantly, one that can be followed with relative ease. I have several patients who have started to successfully follow the diet and think it is wonderful. I have also incorporated it into my own lifestyle, as have two other GP colleagues and several members of staff. Huge congratulations on a life-changing broadcast.

Dr. Pete Bridgwood

> I have several patients who have started to successfully follow the diet and think it is wonderful.

Dear Michael,

I watched your *Horizon* program "Eat, Fast, and Live Longer" with some interest and my family and I decided to try the diet that you suggested. I am a GP in my 50s working in North London. My BMI was 29, but I am otherwise healthy, but do very little exercise. I was somewhat skeptical initially but have managed to lose 13¼ pounds in six weeks and find the diet very simple and easy to follow. I can see no reason why I would not continue in this way for many years. I have presented a summary of your program to a few colleagues and have started to recommend it to some of my patients with startling results.

One particular patient who obviously has metabolic syndrome and a family history of type 2 diabetes had a fasting glucose of 7.2. After only a few weeks, his fasting glucose dropped to 5.9 and he lost 11 pounds. I would like to spread the word even further and wondered if you had plans to design a simple leaflet or website that I could either give to my patients or direct them to view on the Internet. I have difficulty explaining the diet in the short time at the end of one of my 10-minute consultations. I think that this type of manageable eating plan is likely to be so much more successful in managing the obesity epidemic than the current plans to "traffic light" and give fat and sugar contents on food packaging. I think it would be so much more useful to emphasize the calorie content of foods.

Dr. Jon Brewerton

Dear Dr. Mosley,

I watched your original program "Eat, Fast, and Live Longer" on BBC iPlayer in early August. It made good sense to me and I persuaded my husband to watch it, too. Since then we have been following the fasting schedule (with 500 cals for me and 600 for him) most weeks but not every week as sometimes we are only able to fit in one fast a week. Our main motivation is genetically we "could" live fairly long lives. We want those lives to be as healthy as possible.

So far, we have both lost weight (16 pounds for me and 12 pounds for him) and find the fast days fairly easy. And we have both found that we do not overeat on the other days. In fact, I bought a four-finger Kit-Kat for the first time in months yesterday, ate only one finger and put the rest in my bag for later—absolutely unheard of for me as I have struggled with a very "healthy" appetite and have had an unhealthy BMI measurement for most of my life. We have not had our IGF-1 measured, but we are both on high blood pressure medication, and my husband is on high cholesterol medication. We are hopeful that we will see an improvement in these conditions when we next visit our GPs.

I actually find this way of eating much easier than any "diet" I have tried before. I can move the fast days around to cope with our social life.

Yours,

Maureen Johnston

Update from a subsequent e-mail:

As an update, I have now lost 20 lbs and am still finding the whole way of eating easy to do. On our fast days we generally have a cooked breakfast (eggs or oatmeal) and then in the early evening a vegetable-heavy salad in the summer, or vegetable soup in the winter. My husband generally has a slice of bread as his extra 100 cals. We have maintained this way of eating since we saw the original program and expect to continue (possibly with an interruption for Christmas ☺).

Hi, Michael,

I've been doing the intermittent fasting diet for about three months now and wrote a post about it on my blog, *Helena's London Life*.

When I was younger and living in Helsinki I did a few complete fasting sessions with my father. This fast would last five days and you were only allowed to drink fruit juices on the first and last days. So I thought I knew what I was getting into.

But this diet, which basically means you eat *less* on two days per week, is much easier. You're allowed 500 calories (600 for men—so unfair!), which when you think about it isn't that bad. And unlike the fasts of my youth, on this one you're allowed to drink coffee! (Coffee is the one thing I cannot give up these days . . .)

I've been doing the fasting for about three months now, and have lost 11 lbs. I feel so much better on it, not only because of the weight loss, but because I seem to have more energy and control over my eating . . . After the initial shock to the system, your stomach actually contracts and you feel less hungry, more aware of how much you eat on any given day, whether it is one of the 2 or one of the 5 days of the week.

> I feel so much better on it, not only because of the weight loss, but because I seem to have more energy and control over my eating.

So here are my 5 tips to successfully do this diet.

1. Do not do consecutive days—it's too hard and I find the second day in a row grueling. And don't do weekends—we tried a Friday and nearly killed each other.

2. Get busy—the more you have to think about something else other than food, the easier it is. I work from home half of the week, so I try to fast

when I'm in the office. And don't watch Nigella
[Lawson] on TV while fasting. She's like a Domestic
Devil to me on one of my two days.

3. Get yourself an app. I use MyFitnessPal, which is a
simple tool to count the calories. And that is all you
need it for, really, so any other means to do that (a
notepad) is equally good. But for those of you, like
me, who love apps, this one also records the foods
you've used, the exercise you take and the weight
you are losing (and predicts what you would lose
in 5 weeks if each day was like the one you've just
recorded).

4. Don't be too hard on yourself. I have missed a
couple of fasting days during the past three months.
Just because you do that, there's no need to throw
in the towel. There's always tomorrow, or next
week!

5. Don't go alone. Doing this with someone is so
much easier. Some weeks, because of schedules, the
[husband] and I have had to do different days, and
it just doesn't work.

As you see, my experiences have been positive. What
I didn't mention on my blog is that my husband has high
cholesterol, which is an inherited condition, and the main

reason we went on this diet. He didn't need to lose more than [25 lbs or so] in weight (he's always been a racing snake), so now he makes sure he increases his calorie intake (healthily with homemade smoothies) during the five days.

Best regards,

Helena Halme

Dear Dr. Mosley,

I am now 2 weeks into my 5:2 diet and am already seeing a positive effect on my weight. At my second weigh-in I had lost a total of 5 pounds. Feel noticeably slimmer and happy that I can maintain this for a long time to come.

Stats: 5'10" male
Start weight: 191 lbs.
Week 1: 188 lbs.
Week 2: 186 lbs.

Really enjoyed the program!
Kind regards,

Nick Wilson

A busy mum with three children, I was finding losing weight after my having my youngest child really difficult. It didn't help being constantly surrounded by food and snacks, preparing 3 sometimes 4 meals a day for the family. I enjoy food and socializing so restrictive diets just felt like a chore and a battle of willpower every day, so it was never long before I was back to square one again.

The FastDiet, for me, is a more manageable way to lose weight both physically and emotionally, as it's only 2 days a week of "being good" and sticking to 500 calories. It also fits beautifully round my social life, as the fast days can be flexible, therefore I make sure it's a feast day when I'm out for drinks or meals.

It's also not actually that hard for one day to resist temptation, as I know that the next day I can have a donut or a curry and a few glasses of wine if I really want; and when I do, I enjoy it even more without feeling guilty. The proof is, literally, in the pudding; I have been eating and enjoying them on feast days, but sticking to 500 calories on fast days, I am still losing weight. This works.

> The proof is, literally, in the pudding; I have been eating and enjoying them on feast days, but sticking to 500 calories on fast days, I am still losing weight. This works.

Clare Wilson

Posts from Mumsnet.com

Mumsnet is a British website where parents swap advice.

Unhappyhildebrand

Yesterday I ate really well as although I *can* eat what I like I'm also thinking that I don't want to undo all my hard work. So I did have a bag of potato chips, and I did have pork and apple sausages in cider for dinner with one of my daughter's homemade lemon pies afterward, but I didn't have the ton of crap I normally have in between.

I don't think I find the fast days too hard because of the relatively short tunnel and there being light at the end of it. Am looking forward to a weekend of eating normally though!

I think part of what this plan is getting at is we need to learn it's okay to feel hungry and in fact is an essential part of being slim. I speak as a lifelong overeater—the FULL feeling is so normal to me and I had some weird fear about feeling hungry. Well, guess what—it's not the end of the world. I live in a city with stores everywhere—I can have food at any moment I want, so hunger isn't a sign I'm about to perish or get weak. The last couple of months I've been learning to embrace feeling hungry and being comfortable with that—it's a sign from my body to eat again soon (and hopefully that it is burning fat now), not a sign to be feared.

It IS ok to feel hungry. Immediate death from starvation will not occur.

dontcallmehon

Hi all, just wanted to add that exercising whilst fasting was fine for me, too. I spent an hour at the gym last night and felt good. Did 35 mins on the cross trainer and some weights and didn't feel faint or dizzy. It's amazing how good I feel when fasting actually.

ILoveStripeySocks/Jenni Carlin

My Day 1 yesterday also went brilliantly! I wasn't even ravenous when I woke up this morning, I was able to wait an hour before having some toast & peanut butter—and I struggled to finish it!

I loved the feeling of emptiness in my tummy, and the hunger pangs were also enjoyable at times—is this weird? My whole life I had eaten when I wasn't hungry because I was so scared of having a single tummy rumble. I am weirdly looking forward to my next fast day.

Mondayschild78

I did day one yesterday and am feeling brilliant this morning and full of energy. In the end, I just decided to go as long as I could without food. I drank tea with milk and black coffee and water throughout the day. I had some melon and strawberries at 4:00 p.m. then a full dinner of two vegetarian sausages, one boiled egg, one slice of toast, arugula salad with a bit of balsamic. It tasted so good! But the fasting was easier than expected. Wasn't too hungry and just tried to keep busy during the day.

SpringGoddess

Everyone is doing so well. You can really do anything for a day and with a bit of planning I managed to plug most of my hunger pangs down to a manageable level. Scale was showing a good loss this morning.

Any concerns I had on my exercise performance while fasting were scuppered this morning. I ran my fastest sustained pace ever and that is following a 500 cal fast day with no breakfast, only coffee—I smell fat burning!!!! I feel great and will break the fast properly with lunch today. Next fast day is on Thursday. Good luck to everyone fasting today.

Testimonials

BlueDragonLandlady @MsLupin

@DrMichaelMosley We found felt a bit weak when fasting first few weeks, then adapted and fine now.

Valar Wellbeing @ValarWellbeing

@DrMichaelMosley Thanks! We found the show very inspirational and from what people have tweeted us, lots of others did too. Love your shows!

Stickypippa @Stickypippa

@DrMichaelMosley Thankyou for changing my lifestyle. Converted a bunch of people to ADF/5:2 thanks to u, Horizon and @feedfastfeast FB group

susie white @cottagegardener

@DrMichaelMosley As for me, have been IFasting since yr program, changed my attitude to food/hunger, feel energetic & lost nearly [14 lbs]

@alert_bri

@DrMichaelMosley after 4 months on 5:2, agree with your doc assessment . . . This could change the world. Your book should fuel the revolution.

Calorie Counter

All values are for raw product unless otherwise stated.

FOOD	SERVING SIZE	CALORIES PER SERVING
VEGETABLES		
Artichoke, globe	3½ oz.	24
Arugula	3½ oz.	24
Asparagus	3½ oz.	27
Avocado	3½ oz.	193
Bean sprouts	3½ oz.	32
Beets, unpeeled	3½ oz.	38
Bell pepper, any color	3½ oz.	30
Bok choy	3½ oz.	15
Broccoli	3½ oz.	32
Brussels sprouts	3½ oz.	43

FOOD	SERVING SIZE	CALORIES PER SERVING
Butternut squash	3½ oz.	40
Cabbage, green or red	3½ oz.	29
Carrot	3½ oz.	34
Cauliflower	3½ oz.	35
Celeriac	3½ oz.	17
Celery	3½ oz.	8
Chard, green (Swiss)	3½ oz.	19
Chard, rainbow	3½ oz.	17
Chickpeas, dried	3½ oz.	320
Chicory, curly endive	3½ oz.	19
Collard greens	3½ oz.	33
Corn kernels	3½ oz.	115
Cucumber	3½ oz.	10
Edamame, shelled	3½ oz.	117
Eggplant	3½ oz.	18
Endive	3½ oz.	17
Fennel	3½ oz.	14
Garlic	¼ clove	1
Green beans	3½ oz.	25
Jerusalem artichoke	3½ oz.	73
Kale	3½ oz.	33
Leek	3½ oz.	23
Lentils	3½ oz.	319
Lettuce, Boston	3½ oz.	15
Lettuce, frisée	3½ oz.	18
Lettuce, iceberg	3½ oz.	14
Lettuce, romaine	3½ oz.	16
Mushrooms, cremini	3½ oz.	16
Mushrooms, portobello	3½ oz.	13

FOOD	SERVING SIZE	CALORIES PER SERVING
Mushrooms, shiitake	3½ oz.	27
Mustard greens	3½ oz.	26
Onion	3½ oz.	38
Peas, shelled	3½ oz.	86
Peas, baby, frozen	3½ oz.	52
Potato, white, boiling	3½ oz.	79
Radicchio	3½ oz.	19
Radish	3½ oz.	13
Spinach	3½ oz.	25
Spirulina powder	3½ oz.	374
Sweet potatoes	3½ oz.	93
Tomato	3½ oz.	20
Tomatoes, sun-dried, dry-pack	3½ oz.	256
Turnip	3½ oz.	24
Watercress	3½ oz.	26
Zucchini	3½ oz.	18

FRUITS

Açai berry powder	pinch	5
Apple	3½ oz.	51
Apple-blackberry sauce	3½ oz.	107
Apricot	3½ oz.	32
Banana	3½ oz.	103
Blackberries	3½ oz.	26
Blueberries	3½ oz.	60
Cherries	3½ oz.	52
Clementine, peeled	3½ oz.	41
Cranberries	3½ oz.	42
Dried apple	3½ oz.	310

FOOD	SERVING SIZE	CALORIES PER SERVING
Dried apricot	3½ oz.	196
Dried banana chips	3½ oz.	523
Dried blueberries	3½ oz.	313
Dried cranberries	3½ oz.	346
Dried dates, pitted	3½ oz.	303
Dried figs	3½ oz.	229
Dried mango	3½ oz.	268
Dried prunes	3½ oz.	151
Figs, fresh	3½ oz.	74
Goji berries	3½ oz.	313
Grapefruit	3½ oz.	30
Grapes, green, seedless	3½ oz.	66
Kiwi	3½ oz.	55
Lemon	3½ oz.	20
Lime	3½ oz.	12
Mandarin orange, fresh, peeled	3½ oz.	35
Melon, flesh only	3½ oz.	29
Nectarine	3½ oz.	44
Orange, peeled	3½ oz.	40
Papaya	3½ oz.	40
Peach, fresh	3½ oz.	37
Peaches, canned, in juice	3½ oz.	50
Pear, fresh	3½ oz.	41
Pears, canned, in juice	3½ oz.	37
Pineapple, canned, in juice	3½ oz.	50
Pineapple, fresh	3½ oz.	43
Plum	3½ oz.	39
Pomegranate	3½ oz.	55
Pomelo, peeled	3½ oz.	34

FOOD	SERVING SIZE	CALORIES PER SERVING
Prunes, stewed, in juice	3½ oz.	90
Raisins	3½ oz.	292
Raspberries	3½ oz.	30
Satsuma, peeled	3½ oz.	31
Strawberries	3½ oz.	28
Tangerine, peeled	3½ oz.	39
Watermelon, flesh only	3½ oz.	33
GRAINS & GRAIN PRODUCTS*		
Amaranth grains	3½ oz.	368
Bagel, plain	3½ oz.	256
Barley, pearled	3½ oz.	364
Bread, baguette	3½ oz.	242
Bread, ciabatta	3½ oz.	269
Bread, corn	3½ oz.	311
Bread, gluten-free white	3½ oz.	282
Bread, pita	3½ oz.	265
Bread, pumpernickel	3½ oz.	183
Bread, rye	3½ oz.	242
Bread, soda	3½ oz.	223
Bread, sourdough	3½ oz.	256
Bread, spelt	3½ oz.	241
Bread, whole-grain	3½ oz.	260
Breadsticks	3½ oz.	408
Buckwheat	3½ oz.	343
Bulgur	3½ oz.	334
Cereal, All Bran	3½ oz.	334

* Grains and noodles are uncooked unless otherwise specified; cereals and flours are dry.

FOOD	SERVING SIZE	CALORIES PER SERVING
Cereal, shredded wheat	3½ oz.	345
Cereal, Special K	3½ oz.	379
Cornmeal, white or yellow	3½ oz.	364
Cornstarch	3½ oz.	378
Couscous, instant	3½ oz.	358
Crackers, Ryvita	3½ oz.	350
Croissant, plain	3½ oz.	414
Flour, all-purpose	3½ oz.	361
Flour, rice	3½ oz.	364
Flour, rye	3½ oz.	331
Flour, whole-wheat	3½ oz.	336
Granola	3½ oz.	432
Matzo	3½ oz.	381
Millet	3½ oz.	354
Muesli, Swiss-style, unsweetened	3½ oz.	353
Noodles, buckwheat (soba)	3½ oz.	363
Noodles, instant	3½ oz.	450
Noodles, ramen (dry)	3½ oz.	361
Noodles, rice	3½ oz.	373
Noodles, udon	3½ oz.	352
Noodles, vermicelli	3½ oz.	354
Oatcakes	3½ oz.	440
Oatmeal, instant	3½ oz.	380
Oatmeal, old-fashioned rolled	3½ oz.	363
Oats, steel-cut	3½ oz.	373
Pancakes, no syrup	3½ oz.	208
Pasta, white-flour	3½ oz.	370
Pasta, whole-grain	3½ oz.	326
Quinoa	3½ oz.	375

FOOD	SERVING SIZE	CALORIES PER SERVING
Rice cakes	3½ oz.	379
Rice, arborio	3½ oz.	354
Rice, basmati	3½ oz.	353
Rice, brown	3½ oz.	340
Rice, jasmine	3½ oz.	352
Rice, long-grain white	3½ oz.	355
Rice, short-grain white	3½ oz.	351
Rice, white, converted	3½ oz.	344
Rice, white, long-grain	3½ oz.	355
Spelt, pearled	3½ oz.	314
Tortilla, corn	3½ oz.	235
Tortilla, flour	3½ oz.	307
Triticale	3½ oz.	338
Wheatberries	3½ oz.	326
Wild rice	3½ oz.	353
PROTEIN FOODS		
Bacon, Canadian	3½ oz.	128
Bacon, regular, cooked	3½ oz.	441
Bacon, turkey	3½ oz.	123
Beans, baked	3½ oz.	83
Beans, black, dried	3½ oz.	341
Beans, butter, dried	3½ oz.	270
Beans, flageolet, dried	3½ oz.	279
Beans, garbanzo, dried	3½ oz.	320
Beans, kidney, dried	3½ oz.	311
Beans, lima, dried	3½ oz.	282
Beans, navy, dried	3½ oz.	285
Beans, pinto, dried	3½ oz.	309

FOOD	SERVING SIZE	CALORIES PER SERVING
Beans, soy, dried	3½ oz.	375
Beans, white, dried	3½ oz.	285
Beef burger, cooked	3½ oz.	283
Beef, ground lean	3½ oz.	184
Beef, lean	3½ oz.	116
Beef, stewing	3½ oz.	121
Calamari, battered, frozen	3½ oz.	200
Chicken breast, skinless	3½ oz.	105
Chicken liver	3½ oz.	122
Chicken thigh, skinless	3½ oz.	163
Chickpeas, dried	3½ oz.	320
Chorizo sausage	3½ oz.	451
Duck breast, skinless	3½ oz.	92
Edamame, shelled	3½ oz.	117
Egg whites	3½ oz.	50
Eggs, boiled	3½ oz.	154
Eggs, fried	3½ oz.	177
Eggs, omelet	3½ oz.	173
Eggs, poached	3½ oz.	145
Eggs, scrambled	3½ oz.	155
Fish fillet, battered, frozen	3½ oz.	229
Fish fillet, breaded, frozen	3½ oz.	213
Fish fillets, cod	3½ oz.	80
Fish fillets, sole	3½ oz.	78
Fish, white, steamed	3½ oz.	83
Halibut fillet	3½ oz.	100
Ham, lean	3½ oz.	104
Ham, prepackaged, sliced	3½ oz.	118
Hummus	3½ oz.	303

FOOD	SERVING SIZE	CALORIES PER SERVING
Lamb burger, cooked	3½ oz.	267
Lamb chops	3½ oz.	260
Lamb loin	3½ oz.	231
Lamb sausages	3½ oz.	260
Lamb, ground, lean	3½ oz.	235
Lamb, stewing	3½ oz.	175
Lentils, brown	3½ oz.	297
Lentils, green	3½ oz.	316
Lentils, red	3½ oz.	327
Lentils, yellow	3½ oz.	334
Mackerel fillet	3½ oz.	204
Miso	3½ oz.	131
Mussels, shelled meats	3½ oz.	92
Nuts, almond, ground	3½ oz.	618
Nuts, almonds, whole	3½ oz.	613
Nuts, cashew	3½ oz.	583
Nuts, hazelnuts	3½ oz.	660
Nuts, mixed unsalted	3½ oz.	661
Nuts, peanuts, shelled, unsalted	3½ oz.	561
Nuts, pistachio, shelled	3½ oz.	584
Nuts, walnuts, shelled	3½ oz.	693
Peanut butter, natural	3½ oz.	621
Pork sausage, links, cooked	3½ oz.	319
Pork sausage, patty, cooked	3½ oz.	350
Pork, ground, lean	3½ oz.	140
Pork, lean	3½ oz.	117
Rabbit, boneless	3½ oz.	137
Salami	3½ oz.	352

FOOD	SERVING SIZE	CALORIES PER SERVING
Salmon, farmed fillet	3½ oz.	215
Salmon, pink, canned, in water	3½ oz.	131
Sardines, canned, in water	3½ oz.	179
Sardines, fresh	3½ oz.	165
Scallops	3½ oz.	83
Sea bass fillet	3½ oz.	133
Seeds, chia	3½ oz.	422
Seeds, flaxseed	3½ oz.	495
Seeds, hemp	3½ oz.	437
Seeds, pumpkin, shelled	3½ oz.	590
Seeds, sesame	3½ oz.	616
Seeds, sunflower, shelled	3½ oz.	591
Shrimp, shelled	3½ oz.	69
Tahini (sesame paste)	3½ oz.	658
Tempeh	3½ oz.	172
Tofu	3½ oz.	70
Tuna, canned, in water	3½ oz.	108
Tuna, fresh	3½ oz.	137
Turkey, skinless breast fillet	3½ oz.	103
Vegetarian sausage	3½ oz.	114
Veggie burger	3½ oz.	137
Venison steak	3½ oz.	101

DAIRY & DAIRY SUBSTITUTES

Cheese, blue, sheep milk	3½ oz.	368
Cheese, Cheddar, low-fat	3½ oz.	263
Cheese, Cheddar, regular	3½ oz.	410
Cheese, cottage, low-fat	3½ oz.	72
Cheese, cream, very low-fat	3½ oz.	109

FOOD	SERVING SIZE	CALORIES PER SERVING
Cheese, feta	3½ oz.	276
Cheese, Parmesan, grated	3½ oz.	389
Cheese, ricotta, sheep milk	3½ oz.	134
Cheese, soft, goat	3½ oz.	324
Cream cheese, full-fat	3½ oz.	245
Cream cheese, low-fat	3½ oz.	111
Crème fraîche	4 oz.	400
Milk, 1%	4 oz.	50
Milk, 2%	4 oz.	60
Milk, almond, unsweetened	4 oz.	20
Milk, goat, full-fat	4 oz.	84
Milk, rice	4 oz.	60
Milk, skim	4 oz.	43
Milk, soy	4 oz.	40
Milk, whole	4 oz.	75
Sour cream, full-fat	4 oz.	245
Sour cream, low-fat	4 oz.	160
Whipped cream	4 oz.	411
Yogurt, fruited	3½ oz.	94
Yogurt, Greek-style, plain	3½ oz.	132
Yogurt, low-fat, plain	3½ oz.	66
HERBS & SPICES		
Basil leaves, fresh	pinch	0
Cilantro leaves, fresh	pinch	0
Cinnamon, ground	pinch	3
Cloves, ground	pinch	3
Cumin, ground	pinch	4
Ginger, ground	pinch	1

FOOD	SERVING SIZE	CALORIES PER SERVING
Lemongrass, fresh	pinch	1
Mint leaves, fresh	pinch	0
Nutmeg, ground	pinch	4
Oregano, dried	pinch	3
Paprika	pinch	3
Parsley, fresh	pinch	0
Pepper, ground	pinch	3
Rosemary leaves, fresh	pinch	0
Saffron threads	pinch	3
Sage, dried	pinch	3
Sugar, brown	3½ oz.	375
Sugar, white	3½ oz.	385
Tarragon leaves, fresh	pinch	0
Thyme, dried	pinch	2
Turmeric, ground	pinch	3
Vanilla bean	pinch	3

SOUPS

Beef bouillon	4 oz.	7
Beef pho with noodles	4 oz.	90
Chicken and vegetable broth	4 oz.	7
Chicken noodle	4 oz.	50
Cream of mushroom, made with low-fat milk	4 oz.	70
Fish chowder, with milk	3½ oz.	53
Leek and potato	3½ oz.	53
Lobster bisque	4 oz.	124
Miso	3½ oz.	22
Onion	3½ oz.	45

FOOD	SERVING SIZE	CALORIES PER SERVING
Tomato and basil	3½ oz.	40
Tomato bisque, prepared with water	3½ oz.	35
Vegetable	3½ oz.	45
CONDIMENTS & SAUCES		
Agave syrup	3½ oz.	296
Beef gravy, prepared	3½ oz.	45
Capers, drained	3½ oz.	32
Chutney, tomato	3½ oz.	141
Cornichons	3½ oz.	34
Gherkins	3½ oz.	38
Honey	3½ oz.	334
Jalapeños, pickled	3½ oz.	18
Ketchup	3½ oz.	102
Maple syrup	3½ oz.	265
Mayonnaise, fat-free	2 oz.	44
Mayonnaise, light	2 oz.	180
Mayonnaise, regular	2 oz.	360
Mustard, Dijon	3½ oz.	160
Mustard, English, prepared	3½ oz.	167
Mustard, whole-grain	3½ oz.	159
Nutella	3½ oz.	529
Olives, black, pitted	3½ oz.	154
Orange marmalade	3½ oz.	266
Pesto, prepared	3½ oz.	431
Pickled onions	3½ oz.	36
Pickles, mixed, drained	3½ oz.	20
Salad dressing, balsamic, regular	2 oz.	180
Salad dressing, Caesar, low-fat	2 oz.	190

FOOD	SERVING SIZE	CALORIES PER SERVING
Salad dressing, olive oil & lemon	2 oz.	439
Salad dressing, French, low-fat	2 oz.	58
Salsa, tomato	3½ oz.	68
Sauce, barbecue	2 oz.	120
Sauce, caramel	3½ oz.	389
Sauce, chocolate	3½ oz.	367
Sauce, cranberry	3½ oz.	192
Sauce, hollandaise	3½ oz.	239
Sauce, pasta, tomato and basil	3½ oz.	60
Sauce, pasta, vegetable	3½ oz.	50
Sauce, tartar	3½ oz.	358
Sauce, Worcestershire	2 oz.	60
Soy sauce	2 oz.	28
Sriracha	2 oz.	60
Strawberry jam	3½ oz.	258
Tamarind paste	3½ oz.	142
Vinegar, balsamic	2 oz.	56
Vinegar, red wine	2 oz.	12
Vinegar, white wine	2 oz.	12
FATS & OILS		
Butter	3½ oz.	739
Canola oil	2 oz.	480
Corn oil	2 oz.	480
Flaxseed oil	2 oz.	480
Hemp oil	2 oz.	480
Lard	3½ oz.	899
Margarine	3½ oz.	735
Olive oil	2 oz.	480

FOOD	SERVING SIZE	CALORIES PER SERVING
Olive oil spread	3½ oz.	543
Sunflower oil	2 oz.	480
Vegetable oil	2 oz.	480
Vegetable shortening	3½ oz.	900
DRINKS		
Apple juice	8 oz.	120
Beer, amber	10 oz.	77
Beer, lager	10 oz.	80
Cappuccino, fat-free milk	8 oz.	40
Cappuccino, whole milk	8 oz.	70
Champagne	3½ oz.	84
Coca-Cola	8 oz.	90
Coconut water	8 oz.	80
Coffee, black	8 oz.	0
Coffee, with 2% milk	8 oz.	55
Diet Coke	8 oz.	0
Espresso	2 oz.	0
Gin and tonic	7½ oz.	171
Ginger ale	8 oz.	160
Hot chocolate, low-cal, made with water	8 oz.	72
Hot chocolate, made with water	8 oz.	138
Latte, nonfat milk	8 oz.	65
Latte, whole milk	8 oz.	110
Lemonade	8 oz.	94
Lime juice	2 oz.	16
Macchiato, nonfat milk	8 oz.	5
Macchiato, whole milk	8 oz.	10

FOOD	SERVING SIZE	CALORIES PER SERVING
Milkshake, strawberry	8 oz.	256
Orange juice	8 oz.	110
Pear-apple juice	8 oz.	120
Red wine	5 oz.	122
Smoothie, strawberry-banana	8 oz.	140
Sparkling water	8 oz.	0
Sprite	8 oz.	93
Tea, black	8 oz.	0
Tea, chai, 2% milk	8 oz.	120
Tea, green	8 oz.	0
Tea, herbal	8 oz.	0
Vodka and tonic	9½ oz.	170
Wheatgrass juice, frozen	3½ oz.	17
White wine, dry	5 oz.	121
SAVORY SNACKS		
Cheese and chutney sandwich	3½ oz.	228
Cheese straws	3½ oz.	520
Egg and watercress sandwich	3½ oz.	232
French fries, baked	3½ oz.	260
Ham and cheese sandwich	3½ oz.	288
Hummus	3½ oz.	303
Mixed nuts, roasted, salted	3½ oz.	667
Peanuts, dry-roasted, unsalted	3½ oz.	581
Peanuts, roasted, salted	3½ oz.	621
Pizza, tomato-cheese	3½ oz.	258
Popcorn, air-popped	3½ oz.	385
Popcorn, oil-popped, microwave	3½ oz.	535
Potato chips	3½ oz.	529

FOOD	SERVING SIZE	CALORIES PER SERVING
Roasted eggplant spread/dip	3½ oz.	102
Roasted red pepper spread/dip	3½ oz.	235
Taramasalata	3½ oz.	516
Tzatziki	3½ oz.	137
Tuna salad sandwich	3½ oz.	221
Vegetable chips	3½ oz.	502
SWEETS & DESSERTS		
Apple pie	3½ oz.	262
Baklava	3½ oz.	498
Blueberry muffins	3½ oz.	387
Brownie	3½ oz.	419
Carrot cake, iced	3½ oz.	359
Chewing gum, regular	1 stick	11
Chewing gum, sugar-free	1 piece	5
Chocolate cake, iced	3½ oz.	414
Chocolate chip cookies	3½ oz.	499
Chocolate croissant	3½ oz.	433
Chocolate mousse	3½ oz.	174
Chocolate, Cadbury's Dairy Milk	3½ oz.	525
Chocolate, dark	3½ oz.	547
Chocolate, Green and Black, 70%	3½ oz.	575
Chocolate, Green and Black, 85%	3½ oz.	630
Chocolate, Lindt, 70%	3½ oz.	540
Chocolate, milk	3½ oz.	549
Chocolate, white	3½ oz.	567
Cinnamon-raisin loaf	3½ oz.	280
Coconut, desiccated, unsweetened	3½ oz.	632
Coconut, desiccated, sweetened	3½ oz.	466

FOOD	SERVING SIZE	CALORIES PER SERVING
Crystallized ginger	3½ oz.	351
French apple tart	3½ oz.	265
Ice cream, vanilla, regular	3½ oz.	190
Lemon pound cake	3½ oz.	366
Licorice twists	3½ oz.	325
Marshmallows	3½ oz.	338
Milk chocolate–covered raisins	3½ oz.	418
Oatmeal-raisin cookies	3½ oz.	445
Peppermints, Altoids Strong Mints	3½ oz.	395
Popcorn, caramel	3½ oz.	427
Scone, all-butter, plain	3½ oz.	366
Sherbet, lemon	3½ oz.	390
Shortbread cookies	3½ oz.	523
Sorbet, lemon	3½ oz.	118
Tic Tacs	3½ oz.	391
Tiramisù	3½ oz.	263
Toffee	3½ oz.	459
Yogurt-covered raisins	3½ oz.	447

Acknowledgments

This book would not have been possible without the many scientists who gave so generously of their time and research. They include Dr. Luigi Fontana of Washington University School of Medicine; Professor Mark Mattson of the National Institute on Aging; Dr. Krista Varady of the University of Illinois at Chicago; and Professor Valter Longo, director of the USC Longevity Institute.

A huge thanks to Aidan Laverty, editor of BBC's *Horizon*, who pointed me toward the brave new world of intermittent fasting, and to the entire production team, but especially Kate Dart and Roshan Samarasinghe. I'd also like to thank Janice Hadlow, who was brave enough to first put me in front of the camera and gave me the chance to try new things.

Thank you to Nicola Jeal at *The Times* for her constant ingenuity and support.

Our thanks also go to Rebecca Nicolson, Aurea Carpenter, and Emmie Francis at Short Books, for their hard work and immediate grasp of *The FastDiet*'s life-changing potential.

Notes

Chapter One

1 B. M. Popkin and K. J. Duffey, "Does hunger and satiety drive eating anymore? Increasing eating occasions and decreasing time between eating occasions in the United States," *American Journal of Clinical Nutrition*, 91 (May 2010): 1342–47.

2 M. Mattson and E. Calabrese, "When a little poison is good for you," *NewScientist*, 2668 (August 6, 2008): 36–39.

3 A. J. Carlson and F. Hoelzel, "Apparent prolongation of the life span of rats by intermittent fasting," *Journal of Nutrition*, 91 (1945): 363–75.

4 E. Bergamini, G. Cavallini, A. Donati, and Z. Gori, "The role of autophagy in aging: its essential part in the anti-aging mechanism of caloric restriction," *Annals of the New York Academy of Science*, 1114 (October 2007): 69–74.

5 K. A. Varady, S. Bhutani, E. C. Church, and M. C. Klempel, "Short-term modified alternate-day fasting: A novel dietary strategy for weight loss and cardio-protection in obese adults," *American Journal of Clinical Nutrition*, 90, no. 5 (November 2009): 1138–43. M. C. Klempel, C. M. Kroeger, and K. A. Varady, "Alternate-day fasting (ADF) with a high-fat diet produces similar weight loss and cardio-protection as ADF with a low-fat diet," *Metabolism*, 2013 Jan;62(1):137–43. <http://www.ncbi.nlm.nih.gov/pubmed/22889512>

6 M. N. Harvie et al. Genesis Prevention Centre, University Hospital of South Manchester NHS Foundation Trust, UK. "Intermittent, Low-

191

Carbohydrate Diets More Successful Than Standard Dieting; Possible Intervention for Breast Cancer Prevention." Presentation at the CTRC-AACR San Antonio Breast Cancer Symposium, December 2011.

7 M. Hatori, C. Vollmers, A. Zarrinpar, L. DiTacchio, et al., "Time-restricted feeding without reducing caloric intake prevents metabolic diseases in mice fed a high-fat diet," *Cell Metabolism*, 15, no. 6 (2012): 848–60.

8 K. I. Erickson, M. W. Voss, R. S. Prakash, C. Basak, et al., "Exercise training increases size of hippocampus and improves memory," *Proceedings of the National Academy of Science of the United States of America*, 108, no. 7 (January 2011): 3017–22.

9 V. K. Halagappa, Z. Guo, M. Pearson, Y. Matsuoka, et al., "Intermittent fasting and caloric restriction ameliorate age-related behavioral deficits in the triple-transgenic mouse model of Alzheimer's disease," *Neurobiology of Disease*, 26, no. 1 (April 2007): 212–20.

10 Y. Shirayama, A. C. Chen, S. Nakagawa, D. S. Russell, and R. S. Duman, "Brain-derived neurotrophic factor produces anti-depressant effects in behavioral models of depression," *Journal of Neuroscience*, 22, no. 8 (April 2002): 3251–61.

11 B. Li, K. Suemaru, Y. Kitamura, R. Cui, et al., "Strategy to develop a new drug for treatment-resistant depression—role of electroconvulsive stimuli and BDNF," *Yakugaku Zasshi* (*Journal of the Pharmaceutical Society of Japan*), 127, no. 4 (April 2007): 735–42.

12 N. Halberg, M. Henriksen, N. Söderhamn, B. Stallknecht, et al., "Effect of intermittent fasting and refeeding on insulin action in healthy men," *Journal of Applied Physiology*, 99, no. 6 (December 2005): 2128–36.

13 L. Raffaghello, C. Lee, F. M. Safdie, M. Wei, et al., "Starvation-dependent differential stress resistance protects normal but not cancer cells against high-dose chemotherapy," *Proceedings of the National Academy of Sciences of the United States of America*, 105, no. 24 (June 2008): 8215–20.

14 C. Lee; L. Raffaghello, S. Brandhorst, F. M. Safdie, et al., "Fasting cycles retard growth of tumors and sensitize a range of cancer cell types to chemotherapy," *Science Translational Medicine*, 4, no. 124 (March 7, 2012): 124ra27.

15 F. M. Safdie; T. Dorff, D. Quinn, L. Fontana, et al., "Fasting and cancer treatment in humans: A case series report," *Aging*, 1, no. 12 (December 31, 2009): 988–1007.

16 M. N. Harvie, M. Pegington, M. P. Mattson, J. Frystyk, et al., "The effects of intermittent or continuous energy restriction on weight loss and metabolic disease risk markers: a randomized trial in young overweight women," *International Journal of Obesity*, 35, no. 5 (May 2011): 714–27.

17 Page et al., "Waist-Height Ratio as a Predictor of Coronary Heart Disease Among Women," *Epidemiology*, 20, no. 3 (May 2009): 36–66.

18 J. R. Stradling and J. H. Crosby, "Predictors and prevalence of obstructive sleep apnoea and snoring in 1001 middle-aged men," *Thorax*, 46, no. 2 (February 1991): 85–90.

Chapter Two

1 M. N. Harvie, M. Pegington, M. P. Mattson, J. Frystyk, et al., "The effects of intermittent or continuous energy restriction on weight loss and metabolic disease risk markers: a randomised trial in young overweight women," *International Journal of Obesity*, 35, no. 5 (May 2011): 714–27.

2 H. J. Leidy, M. Tang, C. Armstrong, C. B. Martin, and W. W. Campbell, "The effects of consuming frequent, higher protein meals on appetite and satiety during weight loss in overweight/obese men," *Obesity*, 19, no. 4 (2011):818–24.

A. Astrup, "The satiating power of protein—a key to obesity prevention?" *American Journal of Clinical Nutrition*, 82, no. 1 (July 2005):1–2.

T. Halton and F. Hu, "The effects of high protein diets on thermogenesis, satiety, and weight loss," *Journal of the American College of Nutrition*, 23, no. 5 (October 2004):373–85.

3 C. B. Ebbeling, J. F. Swain, H. A. Feldman, W. W. Wong, et al., "Effects of dietary composition on energy expenditure during weight-loss maintenance," *Journal of the American Medical Association*, 307, no. 24 (June 2012):2627–34.

4 C. E. O'Neil, D. R. Keast, T. A. Nicklas, V. L. Fulgoni III, "Nut Consumption Is Associated with Decreased Health Risk Factors for Cardiovascular Disease and Metabolic Syndrome in U.S. Adults: NHANES 1999–2004," *Journal of the American College of Nutrition*, 30, no. 6 (December 2011):502–10.

E. Ros, L. C. Tapsell, and J. Sabate, "Nuts and berries for heart health," *Current Atherosclerosis Reports*, 12, no. 6 (November 2010):397–406.

5 J. S. Vander Wal, A. Gupta, P. Khosla, and N. V. Dhurandhar, "Egg breakfast enhances weight loss," *International Journal of Obesity*, 32, no. 10 (October 2008):1545–51.

6 Brian Wansink, *Mindless Eating: Why We Eat More Than We Think* (New York: Bantam Books, 2006).

7 M. C. Klempel, S. Bhutani, M. Fitzgibbon, S. Freels, and K. A. Varady, "Dietary and physical activity adaptations to alternate-day modified fasting: implications for optimal weight loss," *Nutrition Journal*, 9 (September 2010):35.

8 T. Mann, A. J. Tomiyama, E. Westling, A. Lew, et al., "Medicare's search for effective obesity treatments: diets are not the answer," *American Psychologist*, 62, no. 3 (April 2007):220–33.

9 "The Myriad Benefits of Intermittent Fasting," *Mark's Daily Apple*, http://www.marksdailyapple.com/health-benefits-of-intermittent -fasting/#axzz2GqEVIcd6.

10 Dom Joly, "I've discovered how to lose weight: fast," *The Independent*, November 11, 2012, http://www.independent.co.uk/voices/com ment/ive-discovered-how-to-lose-weight-fast-8303657.html.

11 K. Van Proeyen, K. Szlufcik, H. Nielens, K. Pelgrim, et al., "Training in the fasted state improves glucose tolerance during fat-rich diet," *Journal of Physiology*, 588, Pt 21 (November 2010):4289–302.

12 Klempel et al., op. cit.

13 C. K. Morewedge, Y. E. Huh, and J. Vosgerau, "Thought for food: imagined consumption reduces actual consumption," *Science*, 330, no. 6010 (December 2010):1530–3.

14 E. E. Mulvihill, J. M. Assini, J. K. Lee, E. M. Allister, et al., "Nobiletin attenuates VLDL overproduction, dyslipidemia, and atherosclerosis in mice with diet-induced insulin resistance," *Diabetes*, 60, no. 5 (May 2011):1446–57.

15 E. E. Mulvihill, E. M. Allister, B. G. Sutherland, D. E. Telford, et al., "Naringenin prevents dyslipidemia, apolipoprotein B overproduc-tion, and hyperinsulinemia in LDL receptor-null mice with diet-induced insulin resistance," *Diabetes*, 58, no. 10 (2009):2198–210.

16 K. Fujioka, F. Greenway, J. Sheard, and Y. Ying, "The effects of grape-fruit on weight and insulin resistance: relationship to the metabolic syndrome," *Journal of Medicinal Food*, 9, no. 1 (2006):49–54.

17 M. Waldecker, T. Kautenburger, H. Daumann, S. Veeriah, F. Will, H. Dietrich, B. L. Pool-Zobel, D. Schrenk, "Histone-deacetylase

inhibition and butryrate formation: Fecal slurry incubations with apple pectin and apple juice extracts," *Nutrition*, 24, no. 4 (April 2008):366–74.

18 A. V. Rao and S. Agarwal, "Role of Antioxidant Lycopene in Cancer and Heart Disease," *Journal of the American College of Nutrition*, 19, no. 5 (October 2000):563–9.

19 J. Karppi, J. A. Laukkanen, J. Sivenius, K. Ronkainen, and S. Kurl, "Serum lycopene decreases the risk of stroke in men," *Neurology*, 79, no. 15 (October 2012):1540–7.

20 S. Moghe, "Blueberries may inhibit development of fat cells," Press Release, Federation of American Societies for Experimental Biology, in *Science Daily*, April 10, 2011.

21 T. Miron, I. Shin, G. Feigenblat, L. Weiner, et al., "A spectrophotometric assay for allicin, alliin, and alliinase: with a chromogenic thiol: reaction of 4-mercaptopyridine with thiosulfinates," *Analytical Biochemistry*, 307, no. 1 (2002):76–83.

22 J. Flood and B. Rolls, "Eating soup will help cut calories at meals," Paper presented at the Experimental Biology Conference in Washington, D.C., April 2007. Available in print as "Soup preloads in a variety of forms reduce meal energy intake," *Appetite*, 49, no. 3 (November 2007):626–34.

23 V. Dewanto, X. Wu, K. K. Adom, and R. H. Liu, "Thermal processing enhances the nutritional value of tomatoes by increasing total antioxidant activity," *Journal of Agricultural and Food Chemistry*, 50, no. 10 (April 2002):3010–4.

24 C. Miglio, E. Chiavaro, A. Visconti, V. Fogliano, and N. Pelligrini, "Effects of different cooking methods on nutritional and physicochemical characteristics of selected vegetables," *Journal of Agricultural and Food Chemistry*, 56, no. 1 (December 2007):139–47.

25 Klempel et al., op. cit.

26 C. P. Herman and D. Mack, "Restrained and unrestrained eating," *Journal of Personality*, 43, no. 4 (1975):647–60.

27 V. Schusdziarra, M. Hausmann, C. Wittke, J. Mittermeier, et al., "Impact of breakfast on daily energy intake—an analysis of absolute versus relative breakfast calories," *Nutrition Journal*, 10 (January 2011):5.

28 A. E. Mesas, L. M. Leon-Muñoz, F. Rodriguez-Artalejo, and E. Lopez-Garcia, "The effect of coffee on blood pressure and cardiovascu-

lar disease in hypertensive individuals: a systematic review and meta-analysis," *American Journal of Clinical Nutrition*, 94, no. 4 (2011):1113–26.

S. Larsson and N. Orsini, "Coffee consumption and risk of stroke: a dose-response meta-analysis of prospective studies," *American Journal of Epidemiology*, 174, no. 9 (September 2011):993–1001.

A. Floegel, T. Pischon, M. M. Bergmann, B. Teucher, et al., "Coffee consumption and risk of chronic disease in the European Prospective Investigation into Cancer and Nutrition(EPIC)–German study," *American Society for Nutrition*, 95, no. 4 (April 2012):901–8.

29 D. T. Kirkendall, J. B. Leiper, Z. Bartagi, J. Dvorak, and Y. Zerguini, "The influence of Ramadan on physical performance measures in young Muslim footballers," *Journal of Sports Science*, 26, Supplement 3 (December 2008):S15–27.

30 K. Van Proeyen, K. Szlufcik, H. Nielens, M. Ramaekers, and P. Hespel, "Beneficial metabolic adaptations due to endurance exercise training in the fasted state," *Journal of Applied Physiology*, 110, no. 1 (January 2011):236–45.

31 M. P. Harber, A. R. Konopka, B. Jemiolo, S. W. Trappe, et al., "Muscle protein synthesis and gene expression during recovery from aerobic exercise in the fasted and fed states," *American Journal of Physiology: Regulatory, Integrative and Comparative Physiology*, 299, no. 5 (November 2010):R1254–62.

32 L. Deldicque, K. De Bock, M. Maris, M. Ramaekers, et al., "Increased $p70^{26k}$ phosphorylation during intake of a protein-carbohydrate drink following resistance exercise in the fasted state," *European Journal of Applied Physiology*, 108, no. 4 (March 2010):791–800. Note: This and the preceding three studies were referenced on the Mark's Daily Apple website, http://www.marksdailyapple.com/fasting-exercise-workout-recovery/.

33 Van Proeyen et al., op. cit.

34 G. Reynolds, "Phys Ed: The Benefits of Exercising Before Breakfast," *New York Times*, Well blog, December 15, 2010, http://well.blogs.nytimes.com/2010/12/15/phys-ed-the-benefits-of-exercising-before-breakfast/?src=me&ref=general.

35 M. A Tarnopolsky, "Gender differences in substrate metabolism during endurance exercise," *Canadian Journal of Applied Physiology*, 25, no. 4 (2000):312–27.

36 S. R. Stannard, A. J. Buckley, J. A. Edge, M. W. Thompson, "Adap-

tations to skeletal muscle with endurance exercise training in the acutely fed versus overnight-fasted state," *Journal of Science and Medicine in Sport*, 13, no. 4 (July 2010):465–9.

37 Klempel et al., op. cit.

38 L. K. Heilbronn, S. R. Smith, C. K. Martin, S. D. Anton, and E. Ravussin, "Alternate-day fasting in nonobese subjects: effects on body weight, body composition, and energy metabolism," *American Journal of Clinical Nutrition*, 81, no. 1 (January 2005):69–73.

39 J. Webber and I. A. Macdonald, "The cardiovascular, metabolic and hormonal changes accompanying acute starvation in men and women," *British Journal of Nutrition*, 71, no. 3 (March 1994):437–47.

40 Heilbronn et al., op. cit.

41 Ibid.

42 Klempel et al., op. cit.

43 Ibid.

Index

My FastDiet Diary

My FastDiet Diary

My FastDiet Diary

_____

_____

_____

_____

_____

_____

_____

_____

_____

_____

_____

_____

_____

My FastDiet Diary

About the Authors

Dr. Michael Mosley did his first degree in politics, philosophy, and economics at Oxford University before doing his medical training at the Royal Free Hospital in London. After passing his medical exam, he joined the British Broadcasting Corporation (BBC) as a television producer. There, he created numerous award-winning science and history documentaries for the BBC and for America's Discovery Channel, TLC, and PBS. Among them was the Emmy-nominated series *The Human Face*, with John Cleese and Liz Hurley, the Emmy Award-winning *Pompeii: The Last Day*, and the Emmy-nominated *Supervolcano*. He also helped create the Discovery Channel's Emmy Award-winning film *Global Warming: What You Need to Know*.

Eat, Fast, Live Longer, Dr. Mosley's documentary that inspired this book, will appear on PBS in April 2013 as part of a new series of his documentaries. For his contributions to medical programming, Dr. Mosley was named Medical Journalist of the Year by the British Medical Association.

Mimi Spencer is a journalist and author. For more than twenty years, she has written features for national newspapers and magazines in the UK, including *The Observer, The Times, Vogue,* and *Harper's Bazaar.* As the fashion editor of the *London Evening Standard,* she won the British Fashion Journalist of the Year Award in 2000, and went on to edit the paper's weekly *ES Magazine.* She has had a column in the *Mail on Sunday* for over a decade, writing for 3 million weekly readers about fashion, beauty, food, lifestyle, diet, and body shape. In 2009, drawing on her personal and career interest in women's attitudes to weight loss, she wrote *101 Things to Do Before You Diet.* Today, she writes regularly on women's issues and lifestyle for the Saturday *Times, Marie Claire, Red,* and other publications. She lives in Brighton, on the south coast of England, with her husband and two children.

For more information, visit www.thefastdiet.co.uk.